REIMAGINE

Your Life • Your Purpose • Your Future

Amy White, LPC

William White, Ph.D.

REIMAGINE

Your Life · Your Purpose · Your Future

Copyright © 2019

Ageless IDEAS

ISBN: 9781799073000

All Rights Reserved. No part of this publication may be reproduced, stored in a retrieval system, or transmitted, in any form or in any means – by electronic, mechanical, photocopying, recording or otherwise – without prior written permission.

Ageless IDEAS Publications

Ageless IDEAS Inc

Butler, Pennsylvania

With exceptions as noted in the text, the bible verses quoted are from the ESV Bible. Permission is as follows: Scripture quotations are from the ESV® Bible (The Holy Bible, English Standard Version®), copyright © 2001 by Crossway, a publishing ministry of Good News Publishers. Used by permission. All rights reserved. May not copy or download more than 500 consecutive verses of the ESV Bible or more than one half of any book of the ESV Bible.

TABLE OF CONTENTS

REIMAGINE: A Departure from Mainstream Culture — 4

FOREWORD — 5

INTRODUCTION — 6

CHAPTER 1 - Building a Strong Foundation — 7

CHAPTER 2 - Relationships — 24

CHAPTER 3 - Knowing, Enjoying, and Serving God — 44

CHAPTER 4 - Finding Your Purpose — 66

CHAPTER 5 - Developing Your Emotional Self — 83

CHAPTER 6 – Fortify Your Body and Brain — 118

CHAPTER 7 – Practical Guidance for Exercise, Nutrition, and Sleep — 138

CHAPTER 8 - Who Are You; Where Are You Going? — 162

RESOURCES WORTH DIVING INTO — 176

ABOUT THE AUTHORS — 179

REIMAGINE
A Departure from Mainstream Culture

Society is filled with persons seeking health and immortality from the quick fix, latest ingredient, gadget, or exercise routine. There is no doubt research has demonstrated in a reliable fashion the significant difference a healthy lifestyle can make on one's longevity. What is missing within and across this multifaceted marketing, business, and personal obsession with health is the true meaning and derivation of health or wellness.

Amy and Bill White have stoked the status quo of what it means to be healthy and how one can seek real health. Their new book, a must read, recognizes the limitations of genes, gender, and age when one is about holistic health built around the spiritual, emotional and physical. Critical to their writing is the fundamental idea that health necessitates a real fullness of life, inner peace, and joy. Most important, however, is the realization that these ingredients to health and wellness are not generated from the earth-bound, but rather are gifts granted to us by God to be experienced, nurtured, and shared with others during our short time on planet Earth.

Bill and Amy have generously communicated a path forward for all of us, one authored and taught by God, and one that when genuinely lived will truly grant eternal health and joy for all.

Paul D. Nussbaum, Ph.D., ABPP
Board Certified Clinical and Geropsychology
Fellow National Academy of Neuropsychology
Adjunct Professor of Neurological Surgery,
University of Pittsburgh School of Medicine
President, Brain Health Center
www.brainhealthctr.com

FOREWORD

Architectural basics dating back to Louis Sullivan in 1896 teaches us that, "form follows function." However, American sculptor Horatio Greenough (1805 – 1852) had coined the phrase prior to Sullivan. In other words, the design of a structure or a statue should be determined by its purpose or function.

Building any structure requires planning, tools, labor, commitment, and time. Building a healthy body or mind or soul requires a lifetime. Today, the bookstores and social media bulge at the seams with blueprints for sculpturing a body, or teaching the mind, or developing spiritual growth. But the resources for building a healthy "Life" are in short supply. In *Reimagine*, Bill and Amy White have provided us with not only the tools, but also the muscle and Spirit to make a lasting commitment to building an abundant and fulfilling life, physically, mentally, emotionally, and spiritually; because God did not intend for these areas to be segmented, but to be united to form the whole person.

> Now may the God of peace himself sanctify you completely, and may your whole spirit and soul and body be kept blameless at the coming of our Lord Jesus Christ. (1 Thessalonians 5:23)

When viewing the human life as a design, not only to adapt but also, to conquer the demands imposed on it, life potential becomes unlimited. Reimagine moves us to and through the doorway of this potential and the joy, adventure, and fulfillment that accompanies it by connecting us to the form, purpose, and process that God designed us to function.

Jon Kolb, M.S.

Jon is an exercise physiologist working as a leader, coach, trainer, public speaker, and college professor. Of his outstanding success as a college and professional athlete, he said, "I do not want this to be the highlight of my life." (By the way, Jon earned four Super Bowl Rings, was inducted into the Oklahoma Hall of Fame, and is considered one of the top Steeler players of all time. He was also the winner of the NFL Strongest Man Competition.)

Jon is the founder and leader of *Adventures in Training With a Purpose,* serving veterans, at-risk children, and adults and children with chronic physical and cognitive challenges.

INTRODUCTION

We've known each other for over 33 years and have been married for 29 of them. This is a second marriage for both of us, and we are blessed to have journeyed well together. We have traversed many roads, navigating some more easily than others. Personally and corporately, we've had successes, failures, roadblocks, and traumatic life events. We've lost people we love and experienced unbearable grief. We've endured life-threatening health issues and felt like the rug was pulled out from under us. We have also enjoyed nine children between us, 24 grandchildren, and two great-grandchildren. Through it all, we've gained a profound appreciation for the value of managing life well. We have also both been privileged to step into the lives of other folks, offering a word of encouragement, direction, or insight into advancing to a higher quality of life. What About You?

> *Where do you find yourself today?*
>
> *Where do you want to be tomorrow?*
>
> *Do you know how to get there from here?*

Perhaps your life is pretty much what you aspire to, but you want to grow and discover new things God has prepared for you. Maybe there is a dimension of life where you fall short and would like some input and guidance. Are you in a people-helping role, seeking to enrich your resources to benefit those you serve? We desire to provide a body of helpful life resources, drawing from Scripture and science considered within the framework of Scripture.

> By wisdom a house is built, and through understanding it is established; through knowledge its rooms are filled with rare and beautiful treasures. (Psalm 24:3-4)

This book is about personal growth but also about moving past ourselves, touching the lives of others, and serving God for who He is, not merely for what is in it for ourselves. We pray that in the following pages, you will encounter valuable life resources on the path of becoming all that God calls you to be and your "rooms are filled with rare and beautiful treasures."

Try to be aware of your personal beliefs, thoughts, and feelings and emotions as you read each chapter. *Why* do you believe what you believe, and *how* do your beliefs affect your behavior and your future outlook? What steps to the future are you considering?

May you prosper and be in good health as you continue your journey,

Amy and Bill

CHAPTER 1

BUILDING ON A STRONG FOUNDATION

MIRRORS

The Coach

Bill: My daughter, Stephanie, was nine years old and had returned home from gymnastics practice. She was unhappy and said, "I am never going back there!" Stephanie recited the coach's address to the team about good nutrition, repeating, "Now some of you are fat!" and named Stephanie and three other young gymnasts.

Stephanie and I talked about mirrors—how people are mirrors. What people say and how they act toward us reflects an accurate or distorted image. Sometimes people are like plate-glass-backed-with-silver mirrors, reflecting a correct picture of us; other times, they are like the mirrors at an amusement park, conveying a distorted image.

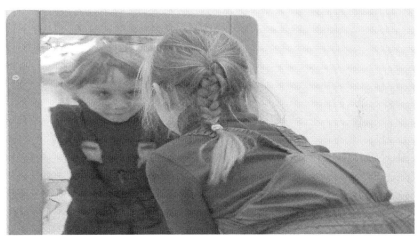

We recalled the fun mirrors she had stood before at Pittsburgh's Kennywood Park. Stephanie realized her gymnastics coach desired the best but had behaved like an amusement park mirror. Stephanie continued her gymnastics, disregarding the coach's well-intended but misguided remarks.

The Bully

One of Bill's childhood mirrors was Dave G, whom Bill refers to as the "honorable bully." Dave was a few years older than Bill and relentlessly teased, threatened, and harassed him. The final straw was the day he tied Bill to a tree in a field and then left the scene.

After Bill freed himself from the ropes, he visited him, saying: "You are older, bigger, and stronger than me." Bill described everything he had done and offered a proposal: "I will wrestle you, and if I win, you have to stop bothering me." Dave agreed and shook Bill's hand to seal the deal. One of Dave's friends served as a witness, and the match proceeded. Bill won with a lucky pin. As the boys stood up, Dave reached out to shake hands and said he would not bother Bill anymore. He kept his word.

Dave's bullying conveyed a negative view of Bill, that he was weak, a victim, and had little value. His handshake and promise kept affirmed Bill and changed Bill's view of Dave. Bill also felt a sense of justice, triumph, of having "clout," leverage, and personal strength – that his choices had made a positive difference.

What About You?

Who and what have been your mirrors, and what have they said about you and life itself? When we embark on a journey of discovery to acquire knowledge and apply wisdom to separate truth from untruth in the mirrors of our experience, we have enormous potential to grow into all we are called to be and live a transformed life.

Each of our life stories has many chapters, some fabulously wonderful and others more challenging, sometimes devastating– all having the potential to educate us and influence us in countless ways. Pain, failure, and suffering are educators, as are love, triumph, and joy. They all matter and help to shape us into who we are. If we are teachable, life is an incredible teacher. Our life experiences are best understood in the context of what is true, derived from a growing understanding of God and the Bible's wisdom.

SETTING THE STAGE

How We Are Made

King David's exclamation, "I am fearfully and wonderfully made!" embraces all humankind worldwide, from our beginning to the present. Our deepest, most central needs issue from how God made us. Each need can be filled only with the substance God created for it.

Consider our multi-dimensional being: God created us with a *spiritual nature*. Only God Himself, in a vital and growing relationship with Him, can satisfy our spiritual nature. We also have a *social nature*, a dimension of our being that can only be filled through enduring, intimate relationships with other people.

We have a *vocational nature*, created to be a self-consistent expression of the unique combination of personality, passion, talents, and aptitudes God has instilled in us. There is a r*ecreative dimension* of our nature—recreation and rest—that contributes to the restoration of body and soul. Our *physical nature* is vitalized through healthy choices informed and confirmed by Scripture and science. We long for closure for things past that continue to impact our life in the present negatively. And on the deepest level of our being, we aspire to *meaningful life*, a sense of *personal dignity*, and *immortality*.

About Our Core Aspirations

We universally share core aspirations for meaning, dignity, and immortality—a drive for a meaningful life, a sense of personal worth based on who we are (not based on our performance or market value), and a means of ultimately circumventing death.

Literature over the ages is filled with affirmations of our search for significance to fulfill our core aspirations. Austrian psychiatrist and Holocaust survivor Viktor Frankl states that at least 20 percent of his patients were suffering from existential neurosis, which has meaninglessness at its roots. He spoke of "the neurosis of our times, the senselessness and aimlessness of people's lives." He says,

> a psychiatrist is confronted more and more with a new type of patient, a new class of neurosis, a new sort of suffering, the most remarkable characteristic of which is the fact that it does not represent a disease in the proper sense of the term . . . I have called this phenomenon which the psychiatrist now has to deal with frequently, 'the existential vacuum.' What I mean thereby is the experience of a total lack, or loss, of ultimate meaning to one's existence that would make life worthwhile.

Philosopher-theologian Dr. Francis Schaeffer underscored our drive for significance and a sense of dignity in his book *No Little People* and a sermon entitled *No Little People, No Little Places.*

C.S. Lewis applies this truth to the significance of our calling: "We may be content to remain what we call 'ordinary people,' but He is determined to carry out a quite different plan. To shrink back from that plan is not humility; it is laziness and cowardice. To submit to it is not conceit or megalomania; it is obedience."

No great friend of religious faith—especially the Christian faith—Sigmund Freud, in Future of an Illusion, asserts religious beliefs are "born of the need to make tolerable the helplessness of man . . . defending himself against the crushing supremacy of nature—earthquake, whirlwind, flood, disease and above all the painful and insoluble riddle of death." In another passage, he says the belief in a future life is "the oldest, strongest, and most insistent wish of mankind."

Some famous philosophers have weighed in as well. The philosopher Georg Wilhelm Friedrich Hegel said, "The highest that has to be transcended is death." Nikolai Berdyaev, the Russian philosopher, says in his autobiography, "I am not prone to the fear of death as, for instance, Tolstoy was, but I have felt intense pain at the thought of death, and a burning desire to restore to life all who have died." Johann Gottlieb Fichte reasons, "Should this life not prove entirely vain and ineffectual, it must at least have relation to a future life, as a means to an end."

We postulate that throughout the earth, from the beginning of human history, all people aspire to a meaningful life, a sense of personal dignity, and immortality—a means of circumventing death. We further postulate that if God is not if God does not exist, life is meaningless, there is no basis for human dignity, and death is not only inevitable but final.

WISDOM

Serious study of Scripture equips us to live wisely. Derek Kidner, in his commentary on the book of Proverbs, says wisdom is "hard won." Wisdom does not drop down from heaven, but it is to be prayed for and pursued with fervor.

What is *wisdom,* anyway? Merriam-Webster defines wisdom as "the natural ability to understand things that most other people cannot understand; knowledge of what is proper or reasonable; good sense or judgment."

Of wisdom, the proverb says, "I love those who love me, and those who seek me find me." (Proverbs 8:17) The Psalmist says, "His delight is in the law of the Lord, and in His law he meditates day and night." (Psalm 1:2) The writer of Psalm 119 says, "Your word I have hidden in my heart, that I might not sin against You. "

To love wisdom is to live it. And wisdom is a means to an end, not the end itself. The ultimate objective of wisdom is to know God intimately and to worship and serve Him.

King Solomon

King Solomon, described in the Old Testament book of First Kings, is famous for his wisdom. God appeared to Solomon during the night in a dream and said to Solomon, "Ask what I shall give you." Solomon's response, "Give your servant an understanding mind to govern your people, that I may discern between good and evil, for who is able to govern your great people?"

> It pleased the Lord that Solomon had asked this. And God said to him, "Because you have asked this, and have not asked for yourself long life or riches or the life of your enemies but have asked for yourself understanding to discern what is right, behold, I now do according to your word. Behold, I give you a wise and discerning mind so that none like you has been before you and none like you shall arise after you. I give you also what you have not asked, both riches and honor so that no other king shall compare with you, all your days." (1 Kings 3:10-13)

> And God gave Solomon wisdom and exceedingly great understanding, and largeness of heart like the sand on the seashore, so that Solomon's wisdom surpassed the wisdom of all the people of the east and all the wisdom of Egypt. For he was wiser than all others . . . and his fame was in all the surrounding nations. (I Kings 4:29-31; McArthur Student Bible Translation)

Many of Solomon's wisdom sayings are contained in the book of Proverbs. Derek Kidner, in his commentary on Proverbs, describes the elements of wisdom as "a rainbow of constituent colors. These all shade into one another and any one of them can be used to represent the whole." Yet he writes that there is some value in "seeing them momentarily analyzed and grouped."

Kidner identifies five synonyms of meaning for wisdom: Wisdom is *instruction* or *training*. It is hard-won and quality of character as much as of mind-. It is, therefore, a matter of discipline. Wisdom is *understanding* or *insight*, the ability to discern good and evil. Wisdom is *wise dealing*, for the fruit is a successful outcome. Wisdom is *shrewdness* and *discretion* with the ability to create and implement plans that result in good. Wisdom is *knowledge* and *learning*, not only information but having an informed mind of knowledge of truth and of God Himself.

Our experiences, the people we encounter, the written materials, and (all too often) the electronic media all shape what we believe, feel, and do. We do well to subject all sources to critical analysis.

Religious sources, such as the Bible, can be scrutinized by answering a few questions: When we do not have the original manuscripts for many religious sources, including the Bible, how are we to know if what we have now corresponds with what was originally written? What does the written document claim or teach with clarity? Can I live out the practical implications of what is taught? Can I live consistently with what a source claims to be true?

Peter S. was having a lively discussion with a college student who claimed, "There is no such thing as good and evil, and physical pain is not real—it is an illusion." In response to that bold claim, Peter tested the denial of evil and pain by gingerly stepping on the young man's foot. The student winced in pain and was indignant in response to the evil Peter had done to him.

In another university setting, John G. conversed with Emil, a student who presented himself as a staunch atheist. The student said, "And if there were a God, I would not want Him to have anything to do with me!" John prayed aloud, "Lord, you have heard what Emil has said. I ask that you have absolutely nothing to do with him." Immediately, Emil blurted, "Stop! Stop! Stop praying that!"

Ask: Is a written source comprehensive as it addresses issues of life; does it provide an adequate basis for answering life's big questions? Is the source accurate as it presents facts and historical events?

Sources of Knowledge

People across the world, in various religions, look beyond their personal experiences to critical writings that provide their life guide and a source for finding a means of fulfilling their deepest aspirations. For example:

- Mormonism: *Book of Mormon, Doctrine and Covenants,* and *Pearl of Great Price*

- Unification Church: Sources include *Divine Principle*

- Scientology: *Dianetics: The Modern Science of Mental Health*

- Buddhism: *Mahavastu, the Jataka Tales, and the Tripitaka*

- New Ageism: *I Ching*, selected passages from the *Bible*, and various writings on mysticism, astrology, and magic

- Hinduism: *Bhagavad-Gita*, the Vedas, and the Upanishads

- Transcendental Meditation: Hindu Scriptures and the writings by Maharishi Mahesh Yogi

- Islam: *Qur'an* (*Koran*)

- Judaism: *Old Testament* with an emphasis on the first five books (Torah), and the *Talmud* which provides an understanding of the *Torah*

- Christianity: Old and New Testaments of the Bible

Any thinking Christian apologist will emphasize that truth is the goal in one's belief system, and a valid worldview would answer significant life questions. Origins: where did I come from? What gives life meaning? Morality: how do I differentiate good from evil? Destiny: where do I go after I die?

As our foundation and framework, we will draw from the wisdom in the Old and New Testaments and explore life-informing evidence offered by the sciences. Historically, men and women filled with God-inspired wonder have been at the forefront of scientific exploration and thought. Many scholars have pointed out that modern science was born because a Christian frame of reference surrounded it. It has been said that Galileo, Copernicus, Francis Bacon, Kepler, Newton, and other scientists believed a reasonable God created the world. Therefore we could find out the order of the universe by reason.

Astrophysicist Dr. Hugh Ross has noted the number of other astrophysicists who have come to recognize the existence of God. But if all you can see is the steel and concrete of the city built by human hands, the magnificence of creation is hidden, with no apparent need to acknowledge the existence of a Creator God. That is the message of a poem, UNTITLED, by Steve Turner in his book, *Tonight We Will Make Love*, Charisma Books, London, 1974)

> We say there is no God
> > (quite easily)
> when amongst the curving
> steel and glass of our own
> > proud creations
>
> They will not argue.
>
> Once we were told of a
> > heaven
> but the last time we strained
> > to look up
> we could see only skyscrapers
> shaking their heads
> > and smiling no.
>
> The pavement is reality.
>
> We say there is no God
> > (quite easily)
> when walking back through
> Man's concreted achievements
> but on reaching the park
> our attention is distracted
> by anthems of birds coming
> from the greenery.
> We find ourselves shouting
> a little louder now because
> > of the rushing streams.
> Our voices are rained upon by
> > the falling of leaves.
>
> We should not take our arguments
> > for walks like this.
> The park has absolutely no manners.

Werner Heisenberg addressed the issue of the compatibility of religion and science:

> In the history of science, ever since the famous trial of Galileo, it has repeatedly been claimed

that scientific truth cannot be reconciled with the religious interpretation of the world. Although I am now convinced that scientific truth is unassailable in its own field, I have never found it possible to dismiss the content of religious thinking as simply part of an outmoded phase in the consciousness of mankind, a part we shall have to give up from now on. Thus in the course of my life, I have repeatedly been compelled to ponder on the relationship of these two regions of thought, for I have never been able to doubt the reality of that to which they point.

As to a belief in God and scientific endeavors being compatible, Heisenberg said, "The first gulp from the glass of natural sciences will turn you into an atheist, but at the bottom of the glass God is waiting for you."

Futurist Robert Jastrow, NASA scientist, astronomer, and planetary physicist, expressed an interesting thought:

> For the scientist who has lived by his faith in the power of reason, the story ends like a bad dream. He has scaled the mountains of ignorance, he is about to conquer the highest peak; as he pulls himself over the final rock, he is greeted by a band of theologians who have been sitting there for centuries.

In this discussion, we will consider the wisdom of the Bible and the knowledge of what is being revealed in the various sciences. Astrophysicist Dr. Hugh Ross said that God authored two books—the first is the Bible; the second is nature, understood in the light of the Bible, and its mysteries are accessible through careful observation and credible scientific research.

How Are You?

How are you? Our question is more than a greeting as we go our merry way. Are you well? Has your wisdom produced good things in your spiritual life, your relationships, your sexuality, your pursuit of life's meaning and purpose, and physical and emotional self? And, what are your sources of knowledge and wisdom?

Your past experiences and interactions with a myriad of people over many years have significantly impacted how you think, feel, believe, act, and your view of self.

Over the entirety of our lives, we have lived individually and in community. We have been wise and other times not so wise, having made some good decisions but also made some bad decisions. We have reaped the reward of wise choices and the negative consequences of those that were not. And, of course, there are events not of our doing— some bringing joy and gratitude, some bringing pain and heartache.

Throughout the pages to follow, we will explore significant areas of life. We desire that our discussion will provide you with quality life mirrors, affirming the best in who you are and helping you to identify and challenge all that has and continues to convey a distorted image. Consider the following questions and what shapes your answer.

- ✓ How do you view yourself concerning your dignity, your aptitudes, and abilities?

- ✓ What most motivates you to do what you do?

- ✓ What is your overall health?

- ✓ How much say do you believe you have in shaping your future, including your well-being?

- ✓ Who are the special people of your life, and what is the quality of your relationship with each?

- ✓ Are there barriers between you and others that can be torn down?

- ✓ Are there unresolved issues past that continue to negatively your life today?

- ✓ If there are such issues, do you know the path to take to erase them?

- ✓ Who is God and what is your relationship with God?

- ✓ What gives you a sense of purpose?

- ✓ What is your vocation; your vocational profile, including your primary passions, your abilities, and your aptitudes?

- ✓ What is your occupation: your "handle" allowing you to confidently fill in the blank: "I am a _____"?

- ✓ What is your job, the specific duties and place of work?

- ✓ What are the things in life that you absolutely love to do and want to be able to continue to do throughout your life?
- ✓ What you believe, and which beliefs matter most?
- ✓ Why do you believe what you believe, and how did you arrive at those beliefs?
- ✓ What matters most to you in life?
- ✓ What do you know – for sure?
- ✓ Is there such a thing as truth?
- ✓ Are there absolutes for discerning right and wrong?
- ✓ Is there anything in your current life that you want to change?
- ✓ Is there a written source that you consider to be truthful, accurate, and authoritative for your life and faith?

THE BIG PICTURE

Living wisdom is holistic. In a sense, it is about making choices to be healthy on all fronts, encompassing every aspect of our lives—*spiritual life, relationships, sexuality, vocation, recreation, physical and emotional well-being, character development, personality, and core beliefs*. Health is much more a function of our daily choices than our genes, gender, or age. Most live below their health, fitness, performance, quality of life, and longevity potential. We can profoundly change the way we age.

Health

Health is an all-encompassing product of many things. It cannot be reduced to a formula of engaging in regular exercise, eating healthy and restful sleep. These necessary but not sufficient elements of life are intended to equip us for what counts most; to enable us to have the health and energy to do all God calls us to do. The broader scope includes our relationship with God; relationships with the special people of our lives; talents and passions expressed in a vocation, regular recreational activity; truth-based, heart-held core beliefs; and achieving closure for past experiences negatively affecting our present lives. God has built a tremendous recovery potential into our bodies and brains. As we age, we can only do what we train for.

Health is not the absence of disease. It is not the absence of something but rather the presence of something positive. Health is the totality of who you have been created to be. You are physically healthy when all bodily organs and bodily systems are structurally sound, fit, and working in harmony. You are fit when you perform at peak performance in aerobic capacity, movement, flexibility, and muscular strength and power.

You are mentally healthy when you exercise personal freedom unencumbered in all areas of life, consistently choosing and behaving to promote your well-being and the good of others; your feelings and expression of emotion fit your circumstances, and you accurately perceive yourself, your life, and your world.

In spiritual health, we suggest you are spiritually healthy when you have a vital and growing relationship with God, know what you believe, why you believe, and your beliefs are characteristically (even though certainly not perfectly) lived out in all phases and dimensions of your life.

As we continue, we will dive into the wisdom of the Old and New Testament and learn from the continuous wave of contemporary science.

Self-Reflection

Whether life has been what we expected or radically different than the ideal we dreamed of long ago, we can draw from experience and reliable sources of knowledge to reshape and build upon the chapters of our personal stories. We can determine who we are in our relationships with others, the world, and God. We can discover and find the best expressions of our enduring aptitudes, gifts, talents, interests, and passions. We can see the greater purpose for why we are here. We can acquire the knowledge and wisdom to care for ourselves and those God has placed in our lives.

HOW TO GET THERE FROM HERE

Don't Go It Alone!

Our need for other people ranges from circumstances in which we are utterly helpless to when we combine our efforts with the talents and energy of others for good. Consider, with gratitude, those who have extended their helping hands and possibly an instance when you were in a situation where you were completely helpless and dependent on another. Let's look at examples that reflect both sets of circumstances.

Shaniqua

Consider the helplessness of eighteen-month Shaniqua Boone dangling four stories above a sidewalk in New York, clutching a curtain. Then she lost her grasp and fell! Quick-acting Keith Manigault, a Wall Street messenger who happened along at the time, ran and broke her fall with his outstretched arms.

Bruce

Dr. Bruce Bickel is a graduate of the Naval Academy, was a quarterback on the Midshipmen's football team, and is the founder and president of Transformational Leadership Group in Pittsburgh. He recounted when he was flying a Navy combat mission during the Vietnam War, and the enemy shot down his aircraft. Badly injured, Bruce activated his landing transmitter and did what he could to stabilize his injuries. Three thousand Vietnamese troops were situated just two hundred yards away. He could hear the enemy cutting a dense jungle path to reach him. Almost two hours later, when his adversaries were yards away, an Air Force Jolly Green Giant rescue helicopter appeared overhead and cleared a chute to the crash site with a six-foot double-blade jungle penetrator.

A rescue paramedic with the call sign "Ice Man" dropped down through the opening, and, seeing Bruce was a Naval officer, he quipped, "If I had known you were an Anchor Clanker, I would not have come down the chute." Bruce retorted: "Son, this is not the best time to be funny." Ice Man, with a calm demeanor and a toothpick in his mouth, gave the reassuring words, "Don't worry, Sir, we have about a minute."

As they were lifted into the helicopter, the enemy overran the crash site and began shooting up through the opening. No one in the helicopter was hit, and they successfully escaped. Bruce later discovered Ice Man was a Native American from South Dakota who had rescued more downed pilots than anybody in Southeast Asia. Because of the intervening hand of God, Bruce's strength of character, and the courageous rescue paramedic and Air Force rescue pilot who put their lives on the line in Southeast Asia, countless lives continue to be impacted and changed for the good through Bruce's decades of service. (Dr. Bickel told this account in a seminar entitled "Making the Right Decisions in the Heat of the Moment" at the 2006 Christian Management Association National Conference.)

Daniel

In the book of Daniel in the Old Testament, we read of Shadrach, Meshach, and Abednego, who were thrown into the fiery furnace by Nebuchadnezzar:

> Nebuchadnezzar then approached the opening of the blazing furnace and shouted, "Shadrach, Meshach and Abednego, servants of the Most High God, come out! Come here!" So Shadrach, Meshach and Abednego came out of the fire, and the satraps, prefects, governors and royal advisers crowded around them. They saw that the fire had not harmed their bodies, nor was a hair of their heads singed; their robes were not scorched, and there was no smell of fire on them. (Daniel 3:26-27)

God also saved Daniel from the lions:

> When he (King Darius) came near the den, he called to Daniel in an anguished voice, "Daniel, servant of the living God, has your God, whom you serve continually, been able to rescue you from the lions?" Daniel answered, "May the king live forever! My God sent his angel, and he shut the mouths of the lions. They have not hurt me, because I was found innocent in his sight." And when Daniel was lifted from the den, no wound was found on him, because he had trusted in his God. (Daniel 6:20-23)

The dramatic circumstances faced by Shaniqua, Bruce, Shadrach, Meshach, Abednego, and Daniel rendered them helpless and dependent. In each instance, God intervened directly, or an agent of God's providence (Keith and Ice Man) acted on their behalf. All of us encounter situations, great and small, beyond our control. And then there are circumstances in which we find ourselves limited—not completely helpless—but others have stepped into our lives to make a difference.

Bill White

I am so grateful. Except for recent medical advances and the fantastic skill of physicians and their teams whom God has brought into my life, I would not have made it past age 50. I was born with a defect in my heart that surfaced in my adult life and has taken me through two heart surgeries. The first was an open chest operation by Dr. Bartley Griffith in 1987; the more recent was in early 2017 through Dr. Douglas Murphy's wonders of robotic surgery. I have gone from sliding into severe heart failure to being able to live an active life. My cardiologist, Dr. Barry Silverman, paved the way for my second heart surgery. During the follow-up visit, he walked into the exam room with the greeting, "My miracle patient." He suggested that I was enabled to undergo the surgery in the first place and fared so well afterward because of the rigorous physical training I have engaged in over my entire life.

THE POWER TO CHOOSE

Amy White

Many years back, I was going through a difficult time. My world had fallen apart on many fronts due to some poor choices I had made, along with the consequences issuing from the actions of others. At one low point, I had to go to court to appeal to the judge regarding a housing situation. The judge did not rule in my favor. I stood in the courthouse hallway tearful, angry, and feeling unjust. I had been misunderstood, unsupported, and left in what I believed to be a place of helplessness. At the moment, I did not think I had any leverage, control, or ability to move in forward in a positive direction.

At that moment, a man in a suit approached me, an attorney. I didn't know him. He looked right at me and said, "Stop crying. You have too much to do." I was taken aback and initially indignant. How dare he rob me of the moment of self-pity that I so deserved! In short order, he outlined the steps I needed to take to resolve what had happened and reach my goal. I never saw him again, but his input changed the outcome for the positive. He cared enough to make a difference in my life perspective.

Realize we do have choices! Bill asked a class of high school students, "How many of you believe you have a say in shaping your future?" Only one of the thirty-one students raised her hand. One young man stated he would be dead before age twenty-five. Another young guy echoed, "Me too." Various factors and life experiences persuaded thirty young men and women that life happens and we don't get a vote. What can parents, family, community, church, and the school do to turn their thinking in a new direction, to help them see they have real choices that will make a difference in their future?

Bill Milliken

Enter Bill Milliken. In the 1960s, Bill, working with kids on New York's Lower East Side in New York, created the Street Academy. A street academy was housed in a storefront and became a path for children who had dropped out of school to reconnect to a future through education. Bill built trusting relationships and persuaded many young people to give education a chance. A typical conversation with the youths Bill met:

> Bill: "Have you given any thought to going back to school?"
>
> Response: "No man, there is no way I am going back to school."
>
> Bill: "What if it were a different kind of school?"
>
> Response: "What do you mean?"
>
> Bill: "I want you to meet somebody."

Bill would take the prospective student to what was affectionately called The Blue Elephant, a blue-painted storefront "school," and introduce the young person to an exceptional and caring teacher. Many accepted Bill's offer and found the path to a promising future.

Skip ahead to the 70s. Bill formed Cities in Schools in New York City, eventually spreading across the nation as Communities in Schools. In 2018 the 131 CIS organizations and licensees partnered with 2,300 schools, served 1.56 million students, and were assisted by 42,000 volunteers. Their mission is "to surround students with a community of support, empowering them to stay in school and achieve in life." Bill says, "It's relationships, not programs, that change children. A great program creates an environment for healthy relationships between adults and children. Young people thrive when adults care about them on a one-to-one level and when they also have a sense of belonging to a caring community."

Since its inception, relationships built through Communities in Schools have enabled countless children to realize the power of their choices in shaping a promising future. 99% of their students stayed in school; 88% met or made progress toward their academic improvement goals; 93% of their seniors graduated or received a GED. The *Communities in Schools* initiative represents vision, compassion, and relationships at their best.

Your Choices

If you are not already won over, our objective is to challenge your thinking. Your choices can make a positive difference in every significant area of life. We have a say in our physical health, reducing our risk for heart disease, stroke, type 2 diabetes, cancer, and dementia and reversing primary diseases already present. Across the age span, we can maintain physical independence with a strong body and sharp brain. We are free to choose the life and career path consistent with how God has made us. We can engage in restorative recreational expressions. We can wisely choose and develop edifying relationships with others, avoiding the heartache of bad relationship choices. We can discard false core beliefs while embracing the truths that will set us free. We can resolve issues past, burdening us with continuing hurt, anger, fear, guilt, shame, and grief. We can jettison the life-counterproductive behaviors and pursuits. We can pursue God with heart, mind, and soul.

CHAPTER 2

RELATIONSHIPS

THE HEART OF THE MATTER

When people ask Amy to state something about herself that might surprise others, she always tells them she is a triplet; one is identical, the other fraternal. She has had two women who have known her since birth, and they've shared thousands of experiences.

As young adults, they all lived nearby and raised their children together. For all of them, it has been nothing short of wonderful to have been born into this relational setting. While the three sisters would have to admit there have been some head-butting here and there, they never had to work at finding a friend at any point in their entire lives. That's significant because we all need people. In this chapter, we will look more in-depth at the value of relationships and how we can choose wisely and maintain healthy relationships.

WE NEED EACH OTHER

The Folks From Roseto

Malcolm Gladwell writes about the town called Roseto in his book The Tipping Point. He addresses the community's unusual characteristics and the reason behind its uniqueness.

A brief recap: In 1882 ten men and one boy left Italy and set sail for New York. They eventually found their way to a slate quarry in Bangor, Pennsylvania.

In the years that followed, more family members joined, and they built homes and a church and called their town Roseto. In 1896 a dynamic priest took over the church and set up spiritual societies and festivals. He encouraged the townsfolk to plant gardens and gave them seeds and bulbs. The town came to life and prospered. Schools, parks, shops, restaurants, and factories sprang up, making blouses for the garment trade.

Jump to the 1950s. Dr. Stewart Wolf from Oklahoma spent summers on a farm near Roseto. On one such visit, he was invited to give a talk at a medical society and afterward met with one physician. The doctor said, "You know, I've been practicing for seventeen years. I get patients from all over, and I rarely find anyone from Roseto under age sixty-five with heart disease." That was well before the advent of cholesterol-lowering drugs and aggressive measures to stop heart disease. Heart attacks were an epidemic in the US and were the leading cause of death in men under the age of sixty-five.

Dr. Wolf decided to investigate and enlisted the support of his colleagues and students from Oklahoma. They analyzed medical records, took medical histories, and constructed family genealogies. They invited the entire town to be tested. Testing was conducted throughout the summer at the local school.

The results were astonishing to Dr. Wolf. No one under fifty-five had died of a heart attack or showed heart disease. For men over sixty-five, the death rate from heart disease was half that of the US. The death rate from all causes in Roseto was 30-35% lower than expected. There was no suicide, no alcoholism, drug addiction, and little crime. No ulcers, either. People were mostly dying of old age. What was the reason for that phenomenon?

Did their dietary practices from the Old World make them healthier than Americans? They cooked with lard, ate pizza loaded with bad stuff, and ate sweets year-round. 41% of their calories came from fat. They smoked and struggled with obesity.

Could the solution be found in their genes? Perhaps they were from a particularly hardy stock that protected them from significant diseases. But Rosetans living in other parts of the US did not have the same good health as their cousins in Pennsylvania.

Was it explained by the region in which they lived? Perhaps the beautiful foothills of eastern Pennsylvania are good for one's health. The towns closest to Roseto, similar in size, of European ancestry, with hardworking folks, had death rates from heart disease three times that of Roseto.

The Answer

It had to do with relationships!

- People visited one another, chatting in the street, cooking for one another in their backyards, sitting on their porches talking.

- The families were multi-generational, mostly living under one roof. Grandparents were greatly respected.

- The church also had a unifying and calming effect.

- There were twenty-two civic organizations in a town under two thousand people.

- The wealthy were discouraged from flaunting their success and helped the unsuccessful with their failures.

They had created a robust, protective social structure capable of insulating them from the pressures of the modern world. They were healthy because of the strong, enduring relationships they had encouraged and built throughout this town.

When the team presented their results to the medical community, they were met with skepticism. No one was used to thinking about health in terms of community. The team had to get them to realize that culture, friends, and family profoundly affect who we are. We are made for people, to: know, enjoy, and serve one another.

More Evidence

Both scientific research and casual observation highlight the deep need for human contact interaction:

- Infants insulated from regular human contact fail to thrive and soon die.
- Children born prematurely in intensive care, are less prone to infection and fare better developmentally when stroked and touched for significant periods each day.
- Children with inadequate human interaction and contact are more prone to illness and fall behind developmentally.
- Even if surrounded by people day-to-day, adolescents are more at risk for depression and suicidal thought and acts if they feel there is no one they can openly talk with when the need arises.
- Adults isolated from others have a significantly higher all-cause death rate than those who are not isolated from others.
- Christians who lack intimacy with parents and friends in their childhood years are often prone to doubt God's acceptance of them and tend to be unsure of their salvation. Their thinking seems to be: "I haven't experienced the love and intimacy with people I can see and touch, therefore how can I know and be assured of the love of God, whom I can neither see nor touch?"

A British Study

Healthy relationships necessitate choosing wisely. Even our Healthy relationships necessitate choosing wisely. Even our health is impacted by the quality of our relationships. A twelve-year research project in the United Kingdom with 9011 British participants (6114 men and 2897 women) revealed that people who experienced negative aspects of a close relationship had a 34% higher risk of coronary incidents than those who did not. The cause was terrible relationships. The researchers eliminated social position, obesity, hypertension, diabetes, cholesterol levels, smoking, alcohol intake, exercise, and fruit and vegetable consumption. Their conclusion: "Be nicer to one another!" (Dr. Roberto De Vogli of the University College, London, UK, and colleagues reported their findings in the October 8, 2007 *Archives of Internal Medicine* issue.)

A dying father

Bill stood beside his dad's hospital bed. He had been in a deep coma for a week following surgery, and there had been not even the slightest observable response from him. Then the phone rang. It was Susan. Bill's dad had been a loyal friend to her and a grandfather figure to her daughter for many years. Bill was deeply moved when she said, "Heather and I will be going to Heaven because your father shared the good news of Jesus with us."

Susan asked to speak with Bill's dad. Bill said, "Although he is unresponsive, in a deep coma, I will hold the phone to his ear, and you can say whatever is in your heart." Bill could hear her voice but could not discern what she was saying. But as she spoke, his father beamed a big smile, the only response we observed between his surgery and his death.

Interestingly, James Lynch, a specialist in psychosomatic medicine, has said that people in a deep coma show improved cardiovascular response to human contact. Loneliness can kill you. James Lynch claimed social isolation leads to physical and emotional deterioration. "Loneliness is pushing our physical health to the breaking point."

Biblical Perspective

The Bible consistently conveys people do best by participating in a community. God establishes the family as the fundamental unit as the bedrock. Family and community fulfill a need built into the nature of the man and woman as God created them. At one time, anthropologists claimed the family was a more recent development, the product of slow evolution. Claude Levi-Strauss and others have pointed out that the available evidence does not support the theory born of biological evolutionism. He states that anthropologists generally lean toward the view that the family, consisting of a more or less durable union, socially approved, of a man and a woman and their children, is a universal phenomenon in all types of society.

As God provides food and air to nourish our bodies, He relates to our need for people by providing opportunities for community and relationships. These needs cannot be written off or ignored. You have no doubt read some version of the adult-to-child conversation in which a boy says he's lonely. The adult tries to reassure him by reminding him that God loves him and is always with him; therefore, there is no need to feel lonely. The boy responds, "But I need someone with skin on!" Only people can fill the people space God has instilled in us. Only God can fill the God space in us.

Genesis reads, "God formed a man from the dust of the ground and breathed into his nostrils the breath of life, and the man became a living being." This man, Adam, was placed in the perfect setting of the Garden and walked in fellowship with God. Yet God said, "It is not good for the man to be alone. I will make a helper suitable for him."

Adam's response to the woman reflects a need that could only be filled by a peer, an equal, a person in the image of God. We don't know how long he waited for Eve, but his response was enthusiastic, to say the least: "At last, this is bone of my bone and flesh of my flesh." Like Adam, we are incomplete apart from community, apart from vital, growing, intimate relationships with other peers. This is the image of the person conveyed throughout the Scriptures and evidenced in current scientific research.

Really? Are we unfulfilled apart from relationships with other people? How can this be so? After all, is God not sufficient in the life of the Christian? Are the song's words, "Jesus Christ is all I need, all I need," not true? Would you also conclude that the mature believer in his faith does not need physical nourishment or oxygen?

The Apostle Paul

Examine the life of the Apostle Paul to see how important people were to him. In his letter to the Philippians, Paul speaks of Epaphroditus:

> But I think it is necessary to send back to you Epaphroditus, my brother, co-worker and fellow soldier, who is also your messenger, whom you sent to take care of my needs. For he longs for all of you and is distressed because you heard he was ill. Indeed he was ill and almost died. But God had mercy on him, and not on him only but also on me, to spare me sorrow upon sorrow. (Philippians 2:25-27)

What Paul meant to others is evident in the Acts 20 account of his meeting with the Ephesian elders:

> When Paul had finished speaking, he knelt with all of them and prayed. They all wept as they embraced him and kissed him. What grieved them most was his statement that they would never see his face again. Then they accompanied him to the ship. (Acts 20:36-38)

The involvement of Paul in the lives of those he cared about so beautifully stands as a model for us. Paul's deep love for others is reflected in his letters to the young churches. People loved Paul. In Acts, chapter 20, Paul is quoted as saying to his fellow believers in Ephesus, "And indeed, now I know that you all, among whom I have gone preaching the kingdom of God, will see my face no more." (Acts 20:25) As Paul was about to leave, we read the account:

> And when he had said these things, he knelt down and prayed with them all. Then they all wept freely, and fell on Paul's neck and kissed him, sorrowing most of all for the words which he spoke, that they would see his face no more. And they accompanied him to the ship. (Acts 20:36-38)

David

Take note of the friendship and enduring bond between David and Jonathan reflected in these words:

> The soul of Jonathan was knit to the soul of David, and Jonathan loved him as his own soul. Jonathan and David made a covenant because he loved him as his own soul. (1 Samuel 18:1-3)

David and Johnathan later had to part. We get a picture of the depth of their relationship:

> David got up from the south side of the stone and bowed down before Jonathan three times, with his face to the ground. Then they kissed each other and wept together—but David wept the most. (I Samuel 20:41)

Throughout the Scriptures, we see people were made for people. Left entirely to ourselves, we tend to function with diminished strength and greater vulnerability. God intended for us to build lasting, quality relationships. The command says we are to love God with all our heart, soul, and strength and our neighbors as ourselves. The love for neighbor involves more than reaching out to those with material needs; it requires giving of ourselves.Friendship

Most of us recognize the space in our hearts reserved for a best friend—the *most* special person among those we invite into our lives. Following is a letter from a young child to another young child, highlighting our desire, even as adults, to be in that special place of friendship with another.

> Dear Stephanie,
>
> I'm sorry about the fight we had in the morning but I still think you would rather be best friends with Jenny and if thats what you want FIGN!
>
> Just forget about me!! why should I care you dont care about me!
>
> P.S. Do you even know Who I am?
>
> Used to be your best friend,

I. STEPS TO GETTING THERE - <u>Exercise wisdom as you choose to invest yourself in relationships</u>

While it is true our greatest joy in life often comes from relationships,

relationships can also be the source of our greatest pain. To a large degree, it may result from choosing the wrong people in the first place! The idea of selecting relationships is foreign to many people. From childhood on, we are thrown into various contexts where we make friends because they cross our path—in our neighborhood, school, work, or church.

CHARACTER

No doubt, the most potent factor for predicting the quality and longevity of a relationship between two people is their maturity of character. Character is to be understood as a whole—the integration of specific attributes in which each factor impacts the others. For example, could a person who lacks courage or honesty be counted upon for loyalty? The qualities of personal integrity and personal strength make a relationship safe, and adding commitment makes for a lasting relationship. Real love in a relationship cannot rise above the maturity of each person. Love is never safe apart from character and never sure apart from commitment.

Are you considering investing in a relationship for a business partnership, dating, engagement, marriage, or friendship? Are you focused on the person's talent, education, personality, or attractiveness? Are you basing your decision on how that person makes you feel about yourself or them? Have you witnessed that person in action over time on the front lines of multiple real-life situations?

Thoughtfully screen folks you consider admitting to your inner circle. Get to know them. It is impossible to know another through conversation only, even exhaustive discussion. To know a person, we must step out of the conversation in the corner of a room and experience them on the front lines of life in various settings, people, conditions, and circumstances over time. "Whoever walks with the wise becomes wise, but the companion of fools will suffer harm." (Proverbs 13:20)

Consider the following character dimensions, understanding that each is a window into a person's overall character. With each consideration, ask what the implications are for my relationship with someone. Start by responding to the items as they relate to yourself, then turn the focus to another.

Personal Strength

- I am **Courageous** – Fear does not direct my decisions.

- I am **Resilient** - I am able to bounce back from difficult times, defeat, and failure.

- I am **Responsible** - I am able to bear up under the weight of responsibilities.

- I am **Persevering** - I stay with a task until it is completed. I see things through.

- I am **Indomitable** - I stay with a valued task even when faced with great obstacles, challenges, difficulty, or pain.

- I am **Self-Controlled** - I am responsive and not reactive. I don't react on the basis of my feelings. I think things out.

Integrity

- I am **Loyal** - I stand by my friends, even when it is costly or painful.

- I am **Caring** - I have the capacity to feel deeply for others, and I take action to help when it is appropriate.

- I am **Principled** - I do what is right, even if at cost.

- I am **Honest** -
  - *Truthful* - I say I believe to be true.
  - *Reliable* - I say I'm going to do something and <u>do</u> it.
  - *Authentic* - What you see is what you get.

- I am **Balanced** – I devote adequate time and energy to *relationships, vocation, recreation, physical* and *spiritual*. I don't over-invest in one area to the loss in other areas.

- I value **Humility** -
  - I am teachable.
  - I do not see myself as better than others because of my position, possessions, health, appearance, or income.
  - I am accountable to others and to high standards, which help me to maintain a "sane estimate of myself."

We are wise to be attentive to how a person treats others. If you see an individual being hurtful to another person, will you be next? Their destructive behavior toward another, sooner or later, may fall on your head. Set your level of expectation and trust in another based upon the person he/she treats worst. The common error is when we bring one into our inner circle based on his or her attractiveness, politeness, or charming personality. Those criteria by themselves are an insufficient basis for building trust. Sometimes a person with a delightful, charismatic personality eventually emerges as controlling and abusive, or worse.

Accepting Imperfections

We are not saying is that each of us should look for perfect people to be part of our lives! We all know that is not realistic as there are no perfect people. All of us have strengths and weaknesses. There are some people who are analytical, discerning, and to whom we seek out when in need of advice regarding finances, problem-solving, and other important issues. They may not be great at empathy and being warm and fuzzy. Other folks may be caring, loving, sensitive individuals who have a great ability to listen and understand, but might not keep a secret well. We never want to throw the baby out with the bathwater because one is lacking in an area. The goal is to have the eyes to see what you are getting.

Picture a continuum for identifying the impact of relationships:

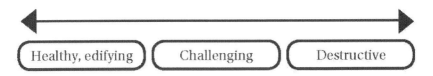

The left side of the continuum refers to folks with whom we can have meaningful but imperfect relationships. They are worth investing in to continue to grow in our relationship with them, even to be part of our inner circle.

The next part of the continuum refers to more challenging people. We may have to do a bit more intensive work in understanding how to manage and relate to these folks. They may be part of our lives, but they would not be good choices to be one of our most trusted friends.

The last part of the continuum recognizes controlling, abusive individuals. We must understand how to identify them, and set good boundaries with them, even if that means cutting them out of our lives altogether.

The primary goal for this type of person is to be in control. They may do so by manipulating our emotions, restraining finances, or physical intimidation or violence. These people may be romantic partners, siblings, coworkers, parents, etc. If you often walk away from an individual feeling wounded or harmed, it is worth exploring if the relationship is abusive and what steps you may need to take to be free from that person.

II. STEPS TO GETTING THERE - **Seek both quantity and quality in relationships**

We live in an age of technology where developing intimate relationships is more challenging. Bill and I went to a restaurant recently. A birthday party was seated at a large table beside us with about a dozen teenage girls. They were all on their phones for a good part of the time, so common these days. Talk about disconnected, non-intimate relationships!

Woody Allen says, "Eighty percent of success is showing up." Showing up—a measure of quantity, not quality—is a necessary condition for a sound, rewarding relationship but not a sufficient condition. The young ladies around the table on their cell phones did show up, but it is only a start.

Ten thousand text messages exchanged between two people is not intimacy. It is not even a path to knowing about those we text with. Even face-to-face conversation, by itself, is insufficient for truly knowing another person. A couple in pre-marriage counseling were asked if they deeply knew one another. They had a standard response, "Oh yes!" When asked to say more about how they had come to know one another so well, they described spending many hours together talking about everything. It is a start.

It has been observed that newly married couples are often unaware of their expectations for one another until they are unmet. A person cannot fully know another by conversing ad infinitum in the confines of a corner of a room.

Making Yourself Known to the Right People and at the Right Time

Through a series of unfortunate events, a successful businessman lost his business, his home, and ultimately his marriage. He hit rock bottom, called several of his friends, and invited them to lunch, all of whom knew of his situation. They each showed up, not knowing why he wanted to meet with them or that the others would be there. Naturally, they were wondering what the deal was.

The host thanked them each for coming and then tearfully shared that he struggled to hold it together. He was afraid he would make unhealthy decisions and then asked them to commit to having a meal with him once a week, either breakfast, lunch, or dinner so that he would connect with at least one person every day. He knew he needed accountability, support, and encouragement and feared what would happen if he did not receive it. That core group, people who knew and loved him, did that. He survived and thrived, returning once again to a place of strength.

The worldwide respected evangelist Billy Graham was once asked if he could go back and live his life again, would he do some things differently? His answer:

Yes, of course. I'd spend more time at home with my family, and I'd study more and preach less. I would not have taken so many speaking engagements, including some of the things I did over the years I probably didn't need to do—weddings and funerals and building dedications, things like that. Whenever I counsel someone who feels called to be an evangelist, I always urge them to guard their time and not feel like they must do everything.

Valuing Others

Taking the time to know others also allows us to pray for them in an up-to-date, intelligent, and specific manner. The concept extends beyond one's family. Consider your world of work. Wayne Alderson gave us some sound advice in his book, Theory R Management, regarding your staff or those in your charge. He describes two types of managers. Which of the two best describes you?

> The first manager places administrative tasks above attending to the people under him/her; the second elevates the people work above the administrative tasks. The traditional manager is expected to say, "I've got to get my paperwork done, no matter what." The people-driven manager says, "I've got to get my people work done, no matter what."

In-depth relationships cannot be built solely in the group or family gathering context. They also require a significant amount of one-on-one time. Paul Tournier, the Swiss psychiatrist, once wrote, "When you add the third person, intimacy is destroyed."

Harry Chapin's song, "Cat's in the Cradle," carries an important message for when we are too busy to spend adequate time with one another. It starts with the words:

A child arrived just the other day; he came to the world in the usual way. But there were planes to catch and bills to pay. He learned to walk while I was away. And he was talkin' 'fore I knew it.

And there is an exchange between father and son:

Son: When you comin' home, Dad?
Father: I don't know when, but we'll get together then. We'll have a good time then, Son. You know we'll have a good time then.

The problem was the son grew up fast, and father and son never did get those special times together. Bill once gave a lecture that he began by playing Harry Chapin's song. In the audience were a couple, a busy pastor and his wife, who had brought their 13-year-old son. As the song's last note sounded, the son jumped to his feet and shouted, "That's my parents!!!"

The parents were red-faced, and the rest of the audience fidgeted uncomfortably in their chairs. These were loving, devoted parents who were over-committed to their work in the community. They were so busy addressing the world's needs that they inadvertently neglected their children and one another.

Community

Charles E. Hummel wrote an essay in 1967 entitled "Tyranny of the Urgent," in which he states many of us are so busy responding to the urgencies of life we don't take time for the important things. One of the important things is spending time with those who mean most to us, with intimacy as an outcome. An instant of intimacy is when two people experience one another at the moment of their happening. It is when people are self-aware and aware of one another while being expressively empathic, honest, and open.

Particular roles and positions, by their nature, lead to isolation. Three come to mind: executives, pastors, and counselors. If you are in this position, you may need to be especially intentional in building relationships.

Our needs, of course, are not all the same. Some of us prefer lots of people in our lives and lots of time with them. Others desire a few good friends they see regularly but don't need to visit daily. No matter the number, we need intimate relationships with those special people. Intimacy has been defined as in-to-me-see, where others know us from the inside out, and we know them similarly. An intimate moment is when two people experience one another, with mutual understanding, in the moment of their happening.

A young woman wrote the following letter to her brother during World War II. It is not profound. It is somewhat mundane, but I'm sure the recipient was delighted with the everyday details shared, given their relationship was characterized by intimacy.

> July 6, 1944
>
> Dear George – Your letter of July 2 was most interesting and I'm glad the candy arrived in good shape. There are more boxes of candy on the way so be prepared. Yes, Hack's letters seem quite cheerful. I drop him a line daily and try to keep him pepped up. Just wrote Clarence again, too. Mother is still doing swell. She received an allotment check for $100 today. She had previously received the $50 initial payment. My checks were $50 each and I received the second one today as she did. I advised her to cash it, because if she returns it, there may be quite a long delay. She will be prepared to refund $50 if necessary. Perhaps they will write in a few days and request it. I'm sure they wouldn't pay for June and then include July in advance. She is standing the heat very well, which means that she is staying close to home. No doubt it is wisest. Tuesday, I worked until 3:00 p.m., had dinner with her, made cookies, and at 9 o'clock walked over to Ruth's for an hour or so, then home. It keeps me busy. Did anyone tell you Lil and Helen were visiting her Monday evening? While they were there Mrs. Gray phoned. I was at Ruth's that day so it seemed as if Thorn Street's former bright lights were all thinking of each other. Guess it will be about the second week in August for you. Hope its sooner. Love – Peg

Peg's brother never made it home. Their many letters became life-long treasures to her.

III. STEPS TO GETTING THERE - **Setting boundaries in relationships**

Boundaries Defined

Relationships fare better when boundaries protect them. To explore the concept of boundaries, let's start with an example. You have saved your money for a long time and are now ready to buy your first home. Your real estate agent takes you to a property that seems perfect. The home's style, layout, condition, and location are exactly what you were looking for, and the price is under your budget! You are feeling excited and ready to make an offer. Before you do, the agent takes you into the backyard. At first glance, it is beautiful! Then you notice something. All your neighbors' backyards to the right, left, and behind seem to be continuous with yours. There are no fences, and now the children who just came home from school run freely across all the properties. You ask the agent about it, and she tells you that part of the HOA agreement is that everyone shares the backyard but reassures you that they all enjoy having everyone around all the time. Do you still think this is the perfect place for you?

Think of boundaries in everyday life as analogous to our property example. Proper boundaries provide a consistent, safe structure for all parties engaged in the relationship, whatever type of relationship it may be, and set reasonable limits on how we invest emotionally, financially, sexually, physically, and in time and energy. Boundaries provide a guide and create protective walls around what we value, whether that is our time, emotions, finances, or ourselves. There is a range of types of boundaries to consider regarding relationships.

Boundaries Related to Our Investment of Time and Energy

Do you feel compelled to say "yes" to the expectations, needs, and requests of others? Do you believe that every need that crosses your path is your responsibility? If you need to please and make people happy—in fact, if you are compassionate, you are more likely to cross boundaries in this area.

A well-known pastor-theologian was asked if we, as caring people, especially those in pastoral or other helping roles, are to martyr ourselves through overworking. After all, there is so much to be done; so many needs. He answered that many folks destroy their health and shorten their lives through overwork, thinking it is serving God. He believed that many running themselves into the ground are not doing God's work in God's way. We are not characteristically called to serve in a manner that will destroy our health.

A guide to setting boundaries in the face of encountering the needs of others is to ask a couple of questions:

- What is to be the division of labor?
- What is my part, what is to be delegated to others, what is the role of the person in need, and what is God's part —that which only He could deliver?

We may be willing to do our part on behalf of others, but we do them a disservice when we do their part for them. (Aside from the fact that we do not have the resources or talent or gifts to meet everyone's needs.) The cast of thousands, other extended community members, may have the necessary skill and resources to address the need. We can work to connect a need to the right persons or resources.

God's Part

Sometimes we are to step back and let a need go painfully unmet till the right person steps in. Think of the typical church setting where only ten percent of the members do all the volunteer work, some of whom think it won't get done if they don't do the work.

Sometimes it is good to leave a void that God will fill in His time. There are needs and circumstances that only God can meet, and we are not God. For example, only God himself can genuinely fill a spiritual void. There is an interesting and relevant brief passage in the book of Ecclesiastes that refers to this dimension of our essential nature:

> He has made everything beautiful in its time. Also, he has put eternity into man's heart, yet so that he cannot find out what God has done from the beginning to the end. (Ecclesiastes 3:11)

Dr. Francis Schaeffer sent a young man back home after being helped while residing in the Swiss L'Abri community for several months. One of the members of the community asked how he could let the man return home when he still had such a long way to grow. He reminded the concerned member that he would not be alone in his journey—God, the Holy Spirit, will be with him every step.

It may be that sometimes we inflate our importance by thinking we have to do it all while diminishing the role of God's spirit in shaping our lives. We can stifle a person's growth by jumping in to help where it is to be left to the power of God or the individual himself. If I carry a person on my back for an extended period, their legs will atrophy. If I take the burden of another, when it is their time to bear it, that person will be stunted in their personal growth.

Yes, there are certainly those times when we are called to take on tasks in the heat of the moment that we are not fully equipped to do. That is not always easy to discern, but we forge ahead to help with God's help. But I delude myself if I think I must come to the rescue in every situation. And there are things that only God can do from the inside out, and in those cases, we are to step back as He does His work. To step in may be to create a dependency on us, underestimate God's role, and inhibit the opportunity for the person in need to step forward and grow.

Discernment

But, you say, how does one know how to distribute the division of labor? How am I to discern my part? The beginning of an answer is to identify the need; explore who has the power, talent, and resources to meet the demand; determine the benefits to be gained or lost by the person in need when he takes decisive action.

As to the cast of thousands, become acquainted with the accessible talents and gifts of others.

As to God's part, study the practical wisdom that flows through the Bible as it addresses the division of labor—for example, the Book of Proverbs in the Old Testament; and the commands and the application of case law of both Old and New Testaments.

As to yourself, embrace all it takes to grow to maturity, and have a sane, humble estimate of your place in the world: neither underestimate nor overestimate who you are.

Boundaries also help us construct a fence around the special people in our lives to ensure adequate and meaningful time together. Let people know they can count on you by showing up for them and being all there when you are with them. How often have we felt that the person we are speaking with is disconnected and preoccupied on their way to something else?

How would you say you are doing in the area of relationships?

Strategies

A. ESTABLISHING A RELATIONSHIP DECISION-MAKING FRAMEWORK. As you carefully consider those you will have in your relational circle, explore the following areas when choosing the special people with whom you develop or maintain relationships.

B. COMMUNICATION

- **Engagement and facilitation.** Volumes have been written about the art of effective communication. It may be productive to explore how well you're doing in the two critical areas discussed below and assess those in your relational circle.

- **Five questions to ask before I speak.** Thoughtful

and productive communication usually comes from operating out of several principles. Consider the following five questions to ask before you speak and evaluating how others are communicating with you – do they work out of a perspective or not?

> **Q 1** Is what I am about to say true?
>
> **Q 2** Will I be understood?
>
> **Q 3** Will my statement accomplish its mission?
>
> **Q 4** Will it promote the best in the other person?
>
> **Q 5** Will it promote the best in our relationship?

Bill met with a guy who was in the doghouse (again). The previous day his wife came home from work announcing that she had gotten another speeding ticket, her third one in a month. He said he exploded, calling her a range of not-so-nice names. Now he was upset with her for being angry with him.

After asking him what he felt when he launched his verbal attack, Bill walked him through the five questions. Responses to the questions are recorded below.

> **Q 1** Are the names you called her an accurate, true description of who she is?

"No, Of course not."

> **Q 2** Were you understood? Given that your obvious goal was to protect your wife from a future accident, did she understand your loving concern?

"No."

> **Q 3** Do you think that your outburst will make your wife a more careful driver?

"Probably not."

> **Q 4** Has your communication over the incident promoted the best, the well-being of your wife?

"No, I guess not."

Q 5   Will this round of negative communication promote the best in your relationship?

"I get the message. I need to apologize to her and describe what I was feeling—my fear—at the time."

The man's angry responses were the secondary emotion. The primary emotion was fear. He was afraid she was at risk for a future accident and was not truly upset about the cost of the fine.

C. <u>DEALING WITH DIFFICULT PEOPLE</u>. As we walk the earth, we will encounter and sometimes deal with folks who are challenging, at least for us. Below are guidelines to consider how to optimally manage these situations.

- <u>Be non-oppositional, non-adversarial</u> (don't argue at every turn; don't declare war. Try to draw out the issue being expressed in a manner that the other person knows you understand, even if you don't agree with their issue or position. Ask questions that facilitate discussion and affirms their value/dignity as a person)

- <u>Be responsive</u> (be non-reactive: consider the other person's frame of reference and the total situation)

- <u>Be connected</u> (be attentive, empathic)

- <u>Be available</u> (Meet him/her on his/her turf, without compromising principle/ integrity).

D. <u>IT IS YOUR TURN.</u> Consider identifying three of the steps you could take within the next week to promote your own knowledge and skill in an area. Pick those that you will do, not necessarily those that you think are most important!

CONCLUSION

At the beginning of the chapter, we mention Amy growing up as a triplet, but there is more to the story. Amy's parents were middle-class and by no means wealthy. They already had three daughters, between 13 and 22 years of age. Their mother was 40 years old, and another pregnancy was not planned. Her mom and dad thought they were almost done raising their family. They were not initially overjoyed with the news that three more children were joining the family, but they managed their assignment well.

They would not know how much these three little girls would be blessed by one another. At age 13, their mom passed away, and their caring and helpful older sisters were out and about raising their children. Their father, while still the responsible parent, was a 53-year-old man grieving the loss of his childhood sweetheart.

The three 'surprises' needed each other in many ways, and their years that followed continued to prove that relationships matter and can contribute to the quality of our lives in immeasurable ways.

We have a social nature, a dimension of our being that can only be filled through enduring, intimate relationships with other people. Our people's space is filled by the face-to-face, flesh, and bones people in our lives.

More from the research

We were created for relationships—a vital and growing relationship with God, and relationships of friendship and family. "Then the LORD God said, "It is not good that the man should be alone; I will make him a helper fit for him." (Gen 2:18)

Harvard conducted a study—the 80-year Harvard Study of Adult Development with the question, "What is the key factor associated with personal happiness, wellness, and longevity?" The answer: Taking the initiative to build close relationships and social connections was correlated with greater happiness and health and greater longevity with a lower incidence of conditions such as type 2 diabetes, dementia, and arthritis. Take note of "taking the initiative to build close relationships," which includes choosing well and investing time and effort to build relationships with others. It is not merely just hanging around other people.

In an article in The New Yorker by Harvard professor Dr. Jill Lapore the U.C.L.A. Loneliness Scale was mentioned. The Scale asks the question,

"Do you often, sometimes, rarely, or never feel these ways?"
> I am unhappy doing so many things alone.
> I have nobody to talk to.
> I cannot tolerate being so alone.
> I feel as if nobody really understands me.
> I am no longer close to anyone.
> There is no one I can turn to.
> I feel isolated from others.

What are your thoughts about the *Lonely Scale*?

CHAPTER 3

KNOWING, ENJOYING, AND SERVING GOD

A SURPRISE ENDING

Dr. David Swanson, the Senior Pastor and Head of Staff at First Presbyterian Church of Orlando, shared the following story in one of his sermons. He began with a prayer: "Lord, we recognize that we know little from our finite human perspective about the spiritual, supernatural world in which you live and abide." He spoke of what he referred to as miraculous moments in our lives that transcend human understanding or definition.

Barbara played the flute in her school band and was active in gymnastics. She continued pursuing these interests throughout her school years but around age sixteen, she started noticing she was tripping over things, bumping into objects, and experiencing a loss of strength in gymnastics practice. She told her parents, and they went to see her family doctor. He referred them to the Mayo Clinic, where Barbara was diagnosed with multiple sclerosis.

While the impact and progression of the disease can vary from person to person, including periods of remission, Barbara experienced a decline over the following 20 years. Her condition compromised her breathing. She was hospitalized occasionally with various infections, her vision deteriorated, and contractures in her hands and feet progressed. Eventually, she was bedridden, a feeding tube was inserted, and she was on supplemental oxygen. The medical staff indicated she may not have long to live. Barbara was moved into hospice care.

But Barbara's story took an incredible turn after a church member called Moody Radio in Chicago implored all the listeners to pray fervently for Barbara. Amazingly, 450 radio audience members sent letters to her church saying they heard the request and were praying.

On Pentecost Sunday, Barbara's aunt and two of her friends visited to encourage her, reading some of the letters sent to the church. Barbara later said that during a lull, she heard a male voice directly behind her say, "My child, get up and walk." Knowing no one was behind her, she believed God was speaking to her. Seeing that she had suddenly become agitated and animated, her friends blocked the opening for her breathing tube so she could talk. She said she believed that God was telling her to get up and wanted her family to be present. Within thirty minutes, they were there.

Barbara removed the covers, removed her oxygen mask, and

stood on legs that had not supported her for eight years. As she stood, she could breathe freely, the contractures in both hands and feet were resolving, and she could feel and use them. Her vision cleared up, and she could identify the people in the room. Her mother got down on her hands and knees, felt Barbara's leg, and told her, "You have muscles!" Everyone in the room began to weep, cry, sing, and pray in praise to God at the miracle before them.

The next day, Sunday, Barbara walked up the aisle of her church in view of everyone, and on Monday, she visited the physician that had been treating her for twenty years. After examining her, he wrote: "I have never witnessed anything like that before, and I consider it a rare privilege to observe the hand of God performing a true miracle."

Barbara's and other experiences like hers raise thought-provoking questions: Did God do that? Does God exist at all? (1.22 billion people consider themselves "nonreligious," including agnostics, atheists, and others who want to remain free from religion per se.) If God does exist, who or what is God? What feelings, positive or negative, were elicited in you by the narrative? Where do we even attempt to begin this exploration?

What do you believe? Why do you believe what you think? My sixth-grade teacher, Miss Garrity, prefaced any challenging task with the words, "Put on your thinking caps." We hope our discussion will stimulate your thinking as we tackle a most challenging topic.

THE SAME GOD?

We live in interesting times. In the minds of many, "Jesus" and "God" do not refer to the Jesus of history or God as He is presented in Scripture, but instead, they refer to Jesus and God in connotation words filled with many different meanings. We do not all believe in the same God.

Examples from Bill

The Professor

In a theological discussion with a university professor, I described God as self-existent, stating:

> I believe if the entire universe—all space, time, matter and energy—were compressed into a tiny ball the size of a pea, and the pea was made to completely disappear, God would still exist. God is the creator of the universe, is quite active in the world and in the

lives of people, but has an independent existence separate from His creation.

The professor countered, "I believe in Gene Hackman's God in the movie, The *Poseidon Adventure*. He said, 'Don't pray to the God out there; look to the God in you.'" What follows is a portion of Hackman's statement from the movie script that the professor alluded to:

> Get down on your knees and pray to God for help? Then everything's going, to work out fine? Garbage! Not where I come from. You can wear your knees off praying for heat in a cold-water flat in February, and icicles will grow on your upraised palms. If you're freezing to death, burn the furniture, set fire to the building, but get off your knees! You know, God's pretty busy. Oh, that doesn't mean that God has forgotten us. On the contrary, he's given to each and every one of us a great and infinite gift, a part of Himself—a spark from His eternal fire to be nurtured within us to keep us warm, to strengthen our efforts. Therefore, don't pray to God to solve your problems—pray to that part of God within you. Have the guts to fight for yourself.

As we continued our discussion, it became clear that the professor's God was in direct contrast with what I described. It could be summed up in two phrases: God is everything; everything is God.

The Student

In a university class lecture, I expressed thoughts about God. Afterward, a student stopped to talk and said he appreciated that I included God in my lecture. As the discussion unfolded, I began to be more specific about the nature of God—who He is and what He is not, just as I had expressed with the professor: If the entire universe—all space, time, matter, and energy—were compressed into a tiny ball the size of a pea, and the pea was made to disappear completely, God would still exist. The student rolled his eyes, lifted his hands, and said, "Oh, I didn't know anyone believed that anymore!" Glancing at his watch, he said, "I've got to go; we can talk later," and hurried away.

The Camper

A high school student said that he felt discouraged. He had attended a weekend camp the prior year and said he had "accepted Jesus into his life." He expected things to change, but being a Christian hadn't made any difference. When asked to describe the anticipated changes, he said he wasn't sure but expected things to improve. I then asked him to explain his view of Jesus. Was he talking about a Jesus who walked on the earth, kicked up real dust as He walked, ate real food, sweat real sweat, bled real blood as he was crucified on a real wooden cross, died, was buried in a real tomb, was raised to life, and is still alive today? His response: "No, I don't believe that!" His responses raise the obvious question: who was the Jesus he had believed in following his previous camp experience?

A Student in Search of Answers to Life's Bigger Questions

An ambitious student was seeking a path for her life, and in this pursuit was launching a study of all the world religions. Such an undertaking would be daunting! There are an estimated 4,000 religions, with four major world religions: Christianity has 2.4 billion adherents; Islam, 1.6 billion; Hinduism, 1.1 billion; and Buddhism, 488 million.

I suggested there is a kind of shortcut for her to consider. All the world's religions have a body of beliefs that can be reduced to a limited number of core or foundational assumptions—called basic presuppositions. Presuppositions, whether they are consciously or unconsciously held, are the bedrock or foundational beliefs that underlie our espoused beliefs, attitudes, opinions, emotions, and feelings. As expressed by Dr. Francis Schaeffer, speaking of the significant number of religions of the world: "When all is done, when all the alternatives have been explored, not many men are in the room."

We all possess deeply-held presuppositions, even if we are unaware of them. Take Dr. Richard L. Rubenstein's assertion, "If there is a God of History, He is the ultimate author of Auschwitz. Therefore, there is no God of History." In his declaration, Dr. Rubenstein implicitly affirms the inherent dignity of persons and the reality of good and evil while denying the existence of God. Yet reason recognizes that the belief in human dignity and the presence of good and evil require the existence of God in the first place. In the words of the character Ivan in Dostoevsky's *The Brothers Karamazov*: "If God does not exist, then everything is permissible."

The Existence of God

Either God exists, or God does not exist. It is gobbledygook to say,

"For you, God exists, but for me, there is no God." And it is more gobbledygook to make up your own god. In the book of Jeremiah, we read:

> A tree from the forest is cut down and worked with an axe by the hands of a craftsman. They decorate it with silver and gold; they fasten it with hammer and nails so that it cannot move. Their idols are like scarecrows in a cucumber field, and they cannot speak; they have to be carried, for they cannot walk. Do not be afraid of them, for they cannot do evil, neither is it in them to do good." (Jeremiah 10:3-5)

For those who love autonomy, or who see God as heavy-handed, the existence of God is a problem. Dr. R.C. Sproul wrote a book entitled, *If There is a God, Why Are There Atheists*? He states there are two reasons why people try to rid themselves of God. The first motive for doing away with God is that we fall short of His standards and stand guilty before him. Nietzsche made the statement: "Man killed God because he couldn't stand to have God looking on his ugliest side. Man must cease to feel guilty."

The second motive for doing away with God is that if He does exist, then we are fully accountable to him. That is, we are under His authority and therefore not the autonomous creatures we desire to be. Author William Braden stated:

> The death of God people are, by and large, a jolly and optimistic lot. This happiness stems from the fact that God is no longer around to spoil the fun, so to speak. (*The Private Sea, LSD and the Death of God*)

A Personal or Impersonal God

If you say God exists, then God is either personal or impersonal. If your working presupposition is that a personal God exists, then in your search, you can eliminate all religions that do not embrace that conviction, such as Buddhism (classical, Zen, Nichiren Shoshu), New Age, Transcendental Meditation, Christian Science, Theosophy, and the Unity School of Christianity, and many others. Religions viewing God as personal include Christianity, Islam, and Judaism.

Self-Existent God?

If God does exist, He is either self-existent or is bound up with the material universe. Either God is self-existent with an existence that is separate from what He has created, or god is everything; everything is god.

Discovering a Path to God

As there are many views of who or what God is, there are also differing views as to the path to God and pleasing him. However, if there is one, personal, self-existent God, *He* will decree how we are to relate to and please Him. He will also have a way of telling us who He is and how we are to reach him. In fact, each religion not only holds a system of beliefs but also a source or sources through which they claim truth is conveyed.

Many religions and their primary (or exclusive) sources of authority were presented in Chapter One. For the Christian Faith, it is the Bible that is authoritative, and the created order conveys something about who God is. As the Apostle Paul states, "His invisible attributes, namely his power and divine nature, have been clearly perceived, ever since the creation of the world, the things that have been made." (Romans 1:20)

The conflicting views espoused in the varied religions of the world are irreconcilable. Where they contradict one another, they cannot be coalesced into a unified view. Will the true religion please stand up?

> **Mormonism:** God was once a man who progressed to become God. He has a physical body. There is no Trinity. God, Father, Son, and Holy Spirit are separate gods. Jesus body was from the sexual union of Mary and Elohim. Salvation is by works, and by being faithful to the leadership.
>
> **Jehovah's Witnesses:** There is one God; no Trinity. Jesus was the archangel, Michael, before he came to earth. Jesus is not God. Eternal life in heaven is by being baptized as a Jehovah's Witness and carrying out their door-to-door efforts in service of their faith.
>
> **Islam:** God is one: There is no Trinity. Jesus, highly regarded, is among one of the 124,000 prophets sent by Allah. Jesus is not God. He was not crucified. Your good deeds, as opposed to bad deeds, determine whether you go to heaven or hell. Paradise includes

maidens to provide sexual pleasure to righteous men.

Orthodox Judaism: God is a spirit, personal, eternal, loving, omnipotent. Jesus is not God. The Messiah eventually will restore the Jewish Kingdom and be the supreme ruler on earth. After a physical resurrection, the obedient will go to heaven; the disobedient will suffer punishment.

New Age: God is not a person; all is god, god is everyone and everything. Jesus is one who drew from the divine power as we all are capable of. He was not the one true God. He did not physically rise from the dead. There is no resurrection of persons; must overcome bad karma with good karma. Reincarnations continue till you achieve oneness with the god who is everything and everyone.

Hinduism: God is a universal spirit, and all of us are a part of god. Jesus is not the one true God but is the son of god in the same sense others are sons of god. He did not rise from the dead, and our sins are not atoned by his death. Many Hindus believe if you have lived a good life, you will be reincarnated into a better life; if you have not lived a good life, you suffer punished through by being incarnated into a life of suffering. It may take many reincarnations, but a goal is to be released from the enduring cycle of rebirths with being in union with Brahma.

Hinduism is multifaceted. It brings together a variety of Indian cultures. Depending on with whom you speak, a Hindu might believe god and all that exists is of one substance, or there are many gods (one tradition says there are 33 million gods), or god abides in trees and rocks, and animals or there is the main god, Brahman, who may take on many forms.

Buddhism: Many view Buddha as a god. Today, many Buddhists in the Western World see Jesus as an enlightened teacher; many of those in the East view Jesus as an avatar, not God. The life goal is nirvana, doing away with all desires. There is an Eightfold Path to eliminating all of life's desires. Included in the eight paths are meditation and right conduct.

In exploring a religion, we do well to consider several factors: its origin, source of authority, view of the nature of God, the path to God, and its anthropology—what it means to be human.

Classical Christianity is summarized in the following Statement of Faith. Compare its core assertions' stark contrast with the various religions of the world.

There is one God, Holy, unchangeable in nature, existing eternally in three persons—the Father, the Son, and the Holy Spirit—each fully and equally possessing all the attributes of God. There is no God before him, or after or beside him. God is a spiritual being, without a physical body.

Jesus Christ, while retaining the fullness of His nature as God, took on a physical body, being miraculously conceived by the Holy Spirit, and born of a virgin. Living a sinless life, He died on the cross to make full payment for our sins, accomplishing salvation once and for all, for all who trust in him alone. He was bodily resurrected; He ascended into heaven. His Deity and perfect humanity are united in one person, forever. He intercedes for us and will return to earth in power and glory.

Humankind was created in the image of God, but because of sin, was alienated from God. That alienation can be removed only through accepting God's gift of salvation through faith alone which was made possible by Christ's atoning death and resurrection. While we are not saved by works, our works are evidence of a new life in Christ.

The Holy Spirit, the third person of the Trinity, convicts us of sin, performs the miracle of new birth, and indwells and empowers believers to live a godly life.

The Bible is God's written, verbally inspired, inerrant revelation to man. It is the ultimate and final authority by which all actions, opinions, beliefs, creeds, and sources of knowledge are to be judged.

GOD AS A PERSONAL BEING

Bill: My son Matthew, age four, and I got into the car to drive to Pizza Hut. Matthew pulled the door shut with both hands, turned toward me with a big grin, and said, "Dad, I like it a lot when only you and I go places together!"

The best gift we have to offer to the special people in our lives is *ourselves*. There is a parallel here between our relationships with others and our relationship with God. Just as Matthew wanted special time with his dad, God desires to have time with each of us. It is almost incomprehensible that THE Mighty God desires a relationship with each of us. He already knows us from the inside out: "This is what the Lord says—he who made you, who formed you in the womb, and who will help you. Fear not . . ." Isaiah 44:2

He wants us to pursue Him:

> Thus says the LORD: "Let not the wise man boast in his wisdom, Let not the mighty man boast in his might, Nor let the rich man boast in his riches; But let him who boasts boast in this, That he understands and knows Me, That I am the LORD, exercising lovingkindness, judgment, and righteousness in the earth. For in these I delight," says the LORD. (Jeremiah 9:23-24)

And what is God's delight? "For I desire mercy and not sacrifice, and the knowledge of God more than burnt offerings." (Hosea 6:6) He wants, and is accessible, to be a part of our lives. It has been said we have a "God-sized vacuum" inside us that only God can fill.

> "There is a sense of eternity in Man's heart which nothing under the sun, but only God can satisfy." (Ecclesiastes 3:11 in the Amplified Bible)

How do we then build an intimate fellowship with the One who made us and who desires our presence? We start in what might first appear to be a difficult place, for we have a problem to solve. The God of Scripture is holy—He is perfection, and we fall terribly short of His standards and what we are created to be.

How do we, falling short of what God requires, come into the presence of the Creator God, who cannot simply overlook sin? The great question of human history is, "How can one who is guilty before a holy God become not guilty?" In the New Testament, Jesus repeatedly claims that He is the way, the door to forgiveness, freedom, and new life: "I am the door. If anyone enters by me, he will be saved and will go in and out and find pasture." (John 10:9)

God provided the solution, a means so amazing and unexpected that no human being could have ever anticipated it. The God of history has a love so great for us that He sent His Son to die to take our place as a payment for our sins. Jesus—fully God, fully man— was the perfect sacrifice. He was the only possible sacrifice to create a bridge for an otherwise unbridgeable chasm. Consider Jesus' saving work in prophecies in the Old Testament and the narratives and doctrinal statements of the New Testament.

> For to us a child is born, to us a son is given, and the government will be on his shoulders. And he will be called Wonderful Counselor, Mighty God, Everlasting Father, Prince of Peace. (Isaiah 9:6)
>
> Long ago, at many times and in many ways, God spoke to our fathers by the prophets, but in these last days he has spoken to us by his Son, whom he appointed the heir of all things, through whom also he created the world. He is the radiance of the glory of God and the exact imprint of his nature, and he upholds the universe by the word of his power. (Hebrews 1:1-3)

God removes our guilt and offers forgiveness, summarized in the whole meaning of the word belief from Jesus' own words in John, chapter three:

> For God so loved the world that He gave His only begotten Son, that whoever believes in Him should not perish but have everlasting life. For God did not send His Son into the world to condemn the world, but that the world through Him might be saved. He who believes in Him is not condemned; but he who does not believe is condemned already, because he has not believed in the name of the only begotten Son of God. (John 3:16-18)

Fortunately, we do not have to earn our way to God. To believe means I acknowledge that Jesus Christ, who is without sin, took my place in satisfying God's justice through his death and resurrection. I accept what he did as "payment in full" for my sin and recognize that His righteousness was "credited to my account." As a follower, I commit to the deepest level of my being to follow Jesus. Walking through this door of faith is the true beginning of a relationship with God.

FAITH

It's a beautiful time of reflection. We have a place where we vacation in the summer. Amy and her family went there when she was a child, she took her girls there, and now they are bringing her grandchildren. Amy's parents are long gone, and there is no family homestead to return to. This place is special for every summer we return home. There is peace, tranquility, and a sense that all is right with the world when we're there.

Faith takes us there in our quest for this same type of eternal destination. And faith is a necessary condition in a relationship with God. "Without faith, it is impossible to please him, for he who comes to God must believe that He is and that He is a rewarder of those who diligently seek him." (Hebrews 11:6)

Faith entails a relationship with God beyond mere intellectual assent to His existence. This thought is carried in the New Testament words, "You believe that there is one God. You do well. Even the demons believe—and tremble!" (James 2:19)

God is much engaged in our lives and the world. He promises that He will be there for us as we continue with him. He will sustain us in the face of the worst of times. You may be a person who has faced imaginable difficulty, pain, or suffering. We could list many who have walked through a corner of hell yet continued to grow in faith, displaying the result of the work of God's Spirit in their lives: love, joy, peace, patience, kindness, goodness, faithfulness, gentleness, self-control. (Galatians 5:22-23)

Faith in the Real World

How would you describe your journey to faith, and the challenges you face? Thoughtfully reflect on the words of educator and writer Nathanael White as he offers a window into his own faith. You might want to read it twice . . . slowly.

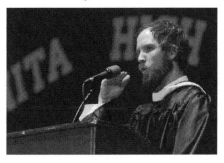

Jonah was commanded by God to tell those in Nineveh that they were sinning and needed to repent. Jonah resisted because he knew that although they were enemy Gentiles, God loved them and would save them. Jonah preferred vengeance so he ran away.

I am my own Nineveh, enemy to myself. I know what I need to do, but, like Jonah, I run. A perpetual prodigal son. I *was* lost, I *was* found, I am lost again. I condemn myself; I love myself; I loathe myself; I long for another self—or maybe just another Earth. Five senses are not enough to know all there is, but is that really what I'm after? The universe is indifferent to my sensing it, but God is not. Then how do I recognize Him?

The object of my faith sits perpetually on the tip of my tongue. It's there, but it's bland and lacks an edge. My words travel the edge of my reach. But I consider this to be some sort of weakness, an inability to commit, some flaw in thinking, bordering on insanity. I need a voice to speak back, tell me everything's going to be okay.

Nonetheless, I pray. But I don't really pray. I'm too old to have quiet time and last time I had quiet time was just after snack time. Now, I eat when I like, but it's much too difficult to pray. I pace. I sit. I stand. I bow. I kneel. I measure what good it will do, what the worthy prayer might be. I need to ask for the right thing, the right way. Otherwise, I'm wasting my time. Need a return on investment.

In spite of it all, He still loves me.

Your Faith Will Be Tested

Meet the Rev. Richard Wurmbrand, who walked through the valley of death. When the communists seized Romania, Pastor Wurmbrand became instrumental in promoting the underground church. His ministry led to him being twice imprisoned for fourteen years, the first three years in solitary confinement, held in a cell thirty feet below ground. Words do not adequately express the suffering he experienced over those years. In solitude, he composed and delivered sermons, painstakingly committing them to memory.

He was frequently pulled out of his cell, tortured, drugged, and then dragged back into his cell. When his memory returned, he continued with his sermons, and by the time of his release, he had composed and memorized 350 of them. His suffering was so great at times he wondered if he was in Hell. He would stare at the cup of water in his cell to reassure himself, thinking, "There is no water in Hell." Add three years to his time in solitary. Rev. Wurmbrand spent five years in a group cell and continued being tortured.

After his release, he continued his work with the underground church for two years, when he was re-arrested and sentenced to twenty-five years. In 1964, five years later, when Norway negotiated with the Communists, Wurmbrand was released. Wurmbrand's knowledge of and relationship with God, a sense of purpose, and incredible personal strength sustained him. God stayed with Wurmbrand, and Wurmbrand remained faithful to God through these long years of suffering.

Can you identify with Wurmbrand? Are there difficult times in your life that have worked for good in the long run? Do you believe God helped you navigate through those times?

Growing in Our Relationship with God

As is true in our people relationships, our relationship with God is nurtured through spending unhurried time, one-on-one with Him, and fellowship with other people. Time with God includes talking with him and thoughtfully meditating on what is written in the Old and New Testaments of the Bible. These are necessary conditions for deepening our knowledge of God and growing in our intimacy with him.

ABOUT THE BIBLE

The literature of the Bible includes parables, wisdom, and poetry. But the Bible also is filled with historical narratives, facts, and witnesses to those facts that demand to be taken seriously. For example, consider Paul's account of those who encountered Jesus after He was resurrected.

> For I delivered to you as of first importance what I also received: that Christ died for our sins in accordance with the Scriptures, that he was buried, that he was raised on the third day in accordance with the Scriptures, and that he appeared to Cephas, then to the twelve. Then he appeared to more than five hundred brothers at one time, most of whom are still alive, though some have fallen asleep. Then he appeared to James, then to all the apostles. Last of all, as to one untimely born, he appeared also to me. (1 Corinthians 15:3-8)

Paul also states, "If in Christ we have hope in this life only, we are of all people most to be pitied."

Some modern minds, even many of those who in the past have taken the Bible seriously, conclude the historical record of Scripture is less than a credible record of the events described. They are being swept along by 21st-century culture. Some seem to believe in a God too small to have pulled off the supernatural events recorded in the Old and New Testaments. And too many folks have stopped thinking. George Bernard Shaw (1856-1950) captured a thought that applies to the 21st-century mindset: "Few people think more than two or three times a year. I have made an international reputation for myself by thinking once or twice a week."

Literature is rated for educational grade level and readability with special analytical tools like the *Gunning Fog Index*. Applying these tools to various texts of Scripture reveals that each writer—Moses, David, Solomon, Paul, Matthew, Mark, John, Luke, Peter, Timothy, etc.—wrote in their unique level, style, grammar, and vocabulary. (For example, the New Testament writers Paul and physician and historian Luke wrote on a higher grade level than John.) God gave us the Bible through human writers, but Scripture reminds us of God's sovereign hand in the writing of the books of the Bible: "All Scripture is breathed out by God and profitable for teaching, for reproof, for correction, and for training in righteousness, that the man of God may be complete, equipped for every good work." (2 Timothy 3:16-17)

> For we did not follow cleverly devised stories when we told you about the coming of our Lord Jesus Christ in power, but we were eyewitnesses of his majesty. (2 Peter 1:16)

> Since I myself have carefully investigated everything from the beginning, I too decided to write an orderly account for you, most excellent Theophilus, so that you may know the certainty of the things you have been taught. (Luke 1:3-4)

> If you call out for insight and raise your voice for understanding, if you seek it like silver and search for it as for hidden treasures, then you will understand the fear of the LORD and find the knowledge of God. For the LORD gives wisdom; from his mouth come knowledge and understanding. (Proverbs 2:3-6)

Historical Evidence

To understand Scripture is to know what we believe and why we believe it, enabling us to present the claims of the Christian faith intelligently. Peter speaks of "always being prepared to make a defense to anyone who asks you for a reason for the hope that is in you." (1 Peter 3:15) Christian books can be helpful (or not), but they should not take the place of a serious study of the Scriptures.

But you might say we do not have the original texts written by these authors. We have copies of copies of copies. We have about a thousand Hebrew manuscripts, including the Dead Sea Scrolls and thousands of manuscript fragments. Of the Greek New Testament, there are 5,800 manuscripts and manuscript fragments. How do we know what was in the originals? The answer is twofold.

First, God promised to preserve the Scriptures: "The words of the LORD are pure words, like silver refined in a furnace on the ground, purified seven times. You, O LORD, will keep them; you will guard us from this generation forever." (Psalms 12:6-7; KJV)

Second, the science of textual criticism (lower criticism, the science of studying ancient manuscripts to determine the authentic text) virtually takes us back to the original writings. There is a small percentage of biblical text in question, but nothing that would bring traditional theology into question.

Modern scholars have studied the books of Luke and Acts regarding the New Testament, finding Luke's historical details are verifiable. A renowned archaeologist, Sir William Ramsey, investigated the Book of Acts beginning with much skepticism. He concluded, "It was gradually borne in upon me that in various details, the narrative showed marvelous truth." Regarding the Old Testament copyists, the scribes were exacting and remarkable in their accuracy. Among the Dead Sea Scrolls was a copy of the book of Isaiah. When it was compared to the one-thousand years later Masoretic text, there was a difference in three words, and they differed only in spelling.

Interpretation

But there is another concern. A common statement about the Bible is that everyone has their interpretations of various texts. You can also get the Bible "to say whatever you want it to say." Others have viewed the Bible as a "living document" that yields different meanings of a text depending on current and cultural practices. The science of hermeneutics—a branch of knowledge that deals with the Bible and other literary texts—yields a reliable interpretation of the writer's intent. Some passages in the Bible are challenging, mysterious, or puzzling:

> Even the archangel Michael, when he argued with the devil and fought over the body of Moses did not dare to bring a slanderous accusation against him." (1 Peter 3:21)

> If anyone sees his brother committing a sin that does not lead to death, he should pray that God would give

> him life. This applies to those who commit sins that do not lead to death. There is a sin that leads to death. I am not telling you to pray about that. (1 John 5:16)

But for the vast majority of Biblical texts, the context and the meaning are quite clear.

Too often, the assumptions (presuppositions) one takes to a text become the basis for interpretation. For example, if one assumes miracles do not occur, a narrative that describes a miracle, such as Jesus' resurrection, is rejected as factual. The first miracle of Jesus turning water into wine is then reinterpreted as follows: Due to the goodwill engendered at the party by Jesus, the host brought out the wine he was holding back. An explanation of how Jesus fed thousands (that occurred at least twice) is that when a little boy shared his five barley loaves and two fish, others were moved to share their food with the crowd. Really? Is your God too weak to perform the miraculous acts recorded in the Bible?

If reading the Bible is new to you, consider beginning your study by reading from the New Testament, the gospel of John, the Book of Acts, and the gospels by the physician Luke, Matthew, and Mark. For a more comprehensive approach, consider reading through the Bible utilizing an approach such as Walk Through the Bible and other sources on the web.

For further study, consider reading:

> *Knowing God*, J. I. Packer (InterVarsity Press, 1993)

> *Classical Apologetics*, R.C. Sproul, Arthur Lindsley and D. John Gerstner (Zondervan, 1984)

Prayer and Meditation

Martin Luther said he spent an hour at the beginning of each day with God—except on very busy days when he spent two hours! Scripture says, "The prayer of a righteous person is powerful and effective" (James 5:6).

If you are new to prayer, it can feel strange, uncomfortable, even daunting. It can help to understand that prayer is having a conversation with God. King David (referred to as a man after God's own heart) in the Book of Psalms speaks often to God. It is beautiful to read his words as he makes himself vulnerable, open, and filled with emotion as he prays. Here is a brief example of the freedom David had to commune with his God:

> Hear my prayer, Lord; let my cry for help come to you.
> Do not hide your face from me when I am in distress.
> Turn your ear to me; when I call, answer me quickly.
> (Psalm 102:1)

Meditation has a variety of definitions, but when we speak about meditation as an expression of Faith, we are speaking of thoughtful devotional contemplation, as is mentioned in the book of Joshua.

> Keep this Book of the Law always on your lips; meditate on it day and night, so that you may be careful to do everything written in it. Then you will be prosperous and successful. (Joshua 1:8)

Jesus taught us about how to pray:

> And when you pray, do not be like the hypocrites, for they love to pray standing in the synagogues and on the street corners to be seen by others. Truly I tell you, they have received their reward in full. But when you pray, go into your room, close the door and pray to your Father, who is unseen. Then your Father, who sees what is done in secret, will reward you. And when you pray, do not keep on babbling like pagans, for they think they will be heard because of their many words. Do not be like them, for your Father knows what you need before you ask him. (Matthew 6:5-8)

Dr. R.C. Sproul suggests using an acrostic guide (ACTS) for our prayer: **A**doration – praise of our creator, savior, loving, all knowing, ever present God. **C**onfession – of our sin, seeking His forgiveness. **T**hanksgiving – having a heart of gratitude for the grace and mercy God has shown to us, and all the blessings he bestows upon us. **S**upplication – bringing our requests to God for ourselves and others. This approach to prayer, with a heart of gratitude, invariably will lead to a renewed understanding and worship of God. It is about Him.

Being Real

We miss the mark when we are less than sincere, honest, and open with God. Of some of the religious people of his day, Jesus said, 'This people honors me with their lips, but their heart is far from me." (Matthew 15:8) We are reminded of some of the great women and men of the Bible who were so honest with God while still showing reverence. Here is a prayer of King David:

> To the choirmaster. A Psalm of David. How long, O LORD? Will you forget me forever? How long will you hide your face from me? How long must I take counsel in my soul and have sorrow in my heart all the day? How long shall my enemy be exalted over me? Consider and answer me, O LORD my God; light up my eyes, lest I sleep the sleep of death, lest my enemy say, "I have prevailed over him," lest my foes rejoice because I am shaken. But I have trusted in your steadfast love; my heart shall rejoice in your salvation. I will sing to the LORD, because he has dealt bountifully with me. (Psalms 13:1-6)

Bill: My daughter, Corrie, then age 7, was tucked in bed, ready to go to sleep when I suggested we pray. She said, "I don't *feel* like praying." I said, it is alright that you don't feel like praying. You can tell God you don't feel like praying and still show your love and respect for Him. She said, "OK, I'll pray!" She then went on to pray the longest prayer I had ever heard from her lips. It began with the gentle words, "Dear Jesus, I don't feel like praying tonight."

Keeping First Things First

I met Auca, a missionary in her seventies, at a leadership conference. Each morning she was by herself in a corner of the lodge, reading and praying. One morning, when she was finished, I walked over and asked how long she had been meeting with God in the morning. She said she had made a commitment at a camp as a teenager to spend the first part of each day with God. Because that was an area of discipline I wrestled with, I asked how she had done over those years. She said, "I've never missed a day."

If I say I love and know another person, but fail to take the time to know, enjoy, and serve them, my words are hollow. Without this one-on-one fellowship with God, no matter how many "spiritual" things we participate in, we become a religious shell.

For Further Study

> *Prayer, Does It Make Any Difference*, Phillip Yancey (Zondervan, 2006)
>
> *The Valley of Vision, A Collection of Puritan Prayers & Devotions* (The Banner of Truth and Trust, 1975)

Also consider utilizing a prayer/meditation/devotional guide such as:

> *My Utmost for His Highest,* Oswald Chambers (Barbour Publishing, Inc., 1963)

Participation in Community

We are made for relationship and community. Worshipping and fellowshipping with others contribute to our personal and spiritual growth. We see a beautiful model of how fellowship took shape in the early church.

> They devoted themselves to the apostles' teaching and to fellowship, to the breaking of bread and to prayer. Everyone was filled with awe at the many wonders and signs performed by the apostles. All the believers were together and had everything in common. They sold property and possessions to give to anyone who had a need. Every day they continued to meet together in the temple courts. They broke bread in their homes and ate together with glad and sincere hearts, praising God and enjoying the favor of all the people. And the Lord added to their number daily those who were being saved. (Acts 2:42-47)

Hebrews 10:25 strongly encourages us not to forsake getting together for worship and fellowship "as is the habit of some." We need each other. Again, going it alone, living on our little island, limits the many good things God intends for us in community with one another.

Some would say they don't need to go to church to worship God. Recent research found people saying, "I love Jesus, but not the church." The church building is not so important; we can gather in a magnificent cathedral or a home church. But we will likely be spiritually undernourished if we withdraw from fellowship and worship with others. Consider visiting a local church or explore joining a small fellowship group or Bible Study. Think about participating in a service group who apply their talents to community needs.

BARRIERS TO KNOWING GOD

Do you have some hesitation? Are you afraid to trust God, to allow

God to speak into your life? Does God love and care about others but not about you? There may be reasons why you have these questions.

A Bad Experience

Amy met with a young woman once who had gone through a horrific experience where she was sexually assaulted. She had nightmares for months, left school, and was getting increasingly isolated from the rest of the world. As she shared her journey, she mentioned meeting with her pastor and others in her church. The advice she received was that she was the problem due to her inability to forgive. Afterward, she wanted nothing to do with the church. Unfortunately, the words of well-meaning people added insult to injury. The young woman was dealing with a myriad of emotions and feelings: injustice, violation, fear, and guilt, among others, that her attacker left her with.

We are all flawed human beings, and the church is not exempt from beliefs and behaviors that cause harm. It's painful to hear and consider the enormous damage that has been done. People sometimes distort the truth, engaging in behaviors "in the name of God" that God has nothing to do with. Jesus taught that His "yoke" is light, and his "burden" is easy. When we build our own "truths," they can be a heavy yoke and an oppressive load to carry. Udo Middleman of L'Abri in Switzerland stated, "Christians have a propensity for adding to the Word of God and binding one another's consciences with what we believe to be right."

The Apostle Paul writes:

> I am astonished that you are so quickly deserting him who called you in the grace of Christ and are turning to a different gospel—not that there is another one, but there are some who trouble you and want to distort the gospel of Christ. But even if we or an angel from heaven should preach to you a gospel contrary to the one we preached to you, let him be accursed. As we have said before, so now I say again: If anyone is preaching to you a gospel contrary to the one you received, let him be accursed. (Galatians 1:6-9)

Relationship Barriers

Our interest in or desire to know God may be diminished because of hurtful experiences in our real-life relationships: parents, dating relationships, coaches, and teachers. For example, you may have a father or mother who treated you harshly, was critical, or even abusive. Perhaps they abandoned or rejected you. It may be difficult to see a heavenly father differently than how you experienced your parent(s). That is understandable. How can you trust a God you cannot see when the one father you did see did not elicit your trust?

Consider the possibility, though, that God may be different than what you imagine. In our human relationships, we trust others based on the evidence they give us that they are trustworthy. Amy: I remember a couple who were struggling. When we got to the root of the problem, the wife was interpreting her husband's behavior as her father's. When he was late, he didn't care about her; when he asked for an alternative food for dinner, she was inadequate. She had to work hard at seeing her husband for who he was, much different from her father. Only then could she accurately interpret his behavior. Trusting God takes time.

A Moment for Reflection

Name the key figures in your growing-up years who were in parenting roles or authority figures, and describe how you have experienced them. Did their behavior toward you influence how you might see God, whom we often see as our heavenly Father?

Unrealistic Expectations

Some would preach a 'name it and claim it gospel—believing in God is a sugar daddy and a means to an end—it's about getting what you want. Others would say if we have enough faith, all illnesses, and woes will be cured. God becomes nothing more than a Fairy Godmother, Santa Claus, or a Genie in a bottle. We are not promised a life devoid of adversity, and we all have areas of vulnerability. If all our dreams do not come true or we succumb to unfortunate circumstances, it is unfair to conclude that God is not with us, does not love us, or that we are less spiritual.

Is Your God Too Small?

When King Solomon dedicated the temple he built to honor God, he said: "But will God dwell on the earth? The heavens, even the highest heaven, cannot contain you. How much less this temple I have built!" (I Kings 8:27)

God is big enough to handle all we struggle with and need—King David certainly didn't hold back. Not only that, God desires that we come to him, place our trust in him, and follow his direction for our lives.

IN SUMMARY

We then refer to important questions that were raised previously: As I live out the wisdom taught in a source, does it promote good or ill for me and for those around me? Does this source provide an adequate basis for answering life's big questions, and for fulfilling core aspirations to meaning, dignity, and immortality?

Our view is that faith is not a blind leap into a belief or religion or worldview. We believe we are to take our brains across the threshold of the door of faith. This is not to deny that there are areas of mystery, but there is a solid case for what we believe and why. There is evidence to satisfy the most brilliant intellect and answer the practical life questions of everyday men and woman.

Three commonly applied tests of truth as it relates to our day-to-day lives: Is it logically sound? Is it supported by the empirical evidence? Will a person thrive if he or she actively lives out that truth in day-to-day life?

There are three tests of truth in a court of law, or in any test of truth: Is it logically consistent? Is there an empirical way to verify what is being asserted? Is there experiential relevance?

As we grow in our relationship with God, over time He transforms us from the inside-out. The fruit of that growing relationship, "love, joy, peace, patience, kindness, goodness, faithfulness, gentleness, self-control." (Galatians 5:22-23) substantially impact our lives and the world around us. These qualities often emerge from the pain and suffering we have endured.

As we engage in an active relationship with God, it is possible that we can experience a level of maturity of character that could only be explained as a result of His continuing activity in our lives. Paul's words to the Christians in Philippi can be applied to us today: "I am confident, that He who has begun a good work in you will complete it until the day of Jesus Christ." It is encouraging to be able to say that one's qualities are attributed to God's work in his/her life. Rather than being dejected about where I fall so short, we celebrate what God has produced in us.

One more reassuring thought: *The God who carries us into this world did not do so to leave us here; when our course is run, our assignment complete, He will also carry us home.*

Now, in the chapter to follow let's consider the quest for our life purpose: what we are called to do and be.

CHAPTER 4

FINDING YOUR PURPOSE

Why are you here? It's easy to be short-sighted as we go through our daily lives, but we don't exist for ourselves. We're an integral part of the bigger picture. God made us exactly the way we are because He has a purpose and calling for our lives. We are most fulfilled when we lose ourselves in One who is much greater than who we are. Fulfilling our purpose includes expressions of our gifts and talents in ways that go far beyond our work and responsibilities. It includes knowing how to make ourselves available to be used by God to make a positive difference as we actively demonstrate His love and help overturn the consequences of a fallen world.

As you explore how to define and express your passions, consider also 'giving yourself away' by using your unique combination of talents and aptitudes as a "specialist volunteer," expanding the length and breadth of your impact on the lives of others.

The Architect

Some years back, Bill spent the summer at L'Abri in Switzerland. As a student, he had the opportunity to present a lecture for critique by the staff and students of the community. After the session, he was approached by a visiting guest, an architect, with his practice in Italy. He said he had come to L'Abri to find answers to troubling life questions. That initial meeting led to a lengthy discussion that evening, an interaction that began in the local pub and then spilled out onto the sidewalk for a couple more hours.

He shared a story about a time when he felt that his life was meaningless, despite his great success as an architect. He had worked out a detailed plan to take his life and proceeded to implement it. He closed the doors to the kitchen, stuffed rags under each door, and turned on the stove gas jets. Then it struck him that his daughter was liable to stop in to visit and would foil his plan. He turned off the gas jets and called her, saying he was unavailable for a few hours, so please don't stop by. Then he reopened the gas jets as planned. His daughter, sensing a troubling tone of his voice, rushed to his house in time to rescue him.

The architect has lots of company in his search for meaning. Like all of us, he aspires to a meaningful life, a quality inherent in being human. Work by itself, even when it is a good fit, can leave us unfulfilled and wandering like lost sheep. Connecting God's purpose with how He made us and our work is a formula for being fulfilled.

WRAPPING OUR BRAINS AROUND
LIFE PURPOSE AND MEANING

A sense of purpose is the reason to get up from bed each day. It is the "why" of living, the driving force that motivates meaningful action. The *foundation* for the meaning of life is in knowing, enjoying, and serving the God of history, the Creator and Sustainer of all that is. On that foundation is built a meaningful life.

RELATIONSHIPS

Parallel with our relationship with God, it is knowing, enjoying, and serving the special people of our lives.

VOCATION (includes avocation)

Expressions of our work are a self-consistent expression of our passions, interests, talents, abilities, and aptitudes. Vocation is our main line of work; avocation is a complementary expression of our talents and passions, typically through tasks lacking in our primary work.

Being **FORTIFIED** in Body and Brain

Recognizing that God has created the amazing body and brain, good bodily stewardship honors God and equips us to serve him in all we are called to do.

Being fortified means that the body and brain's physical structure (physiology) are healthy, sound at the core, and developed to their whole physical well-being. A healthy brain, for example, is much more than the absence of disease. A healthy brain means that all 86 billion neurons and their nourishing blood circulation, brain chemistry, and the cleansing channels of the brain are poised to do all that the brain is supposed to do—to be conscious, to learn, to remember, to focus and concentrate, to problem-solve, to perceive the world accurately, to act constructively, to inhibit actions that are counter-productive or destructive, to enable us to move about, to orchestrate the automatic functions of the body, and to express one's unique personality.

Being fortified is also being enriched so that the body and brain are trained to their highest level of fitness and performance. For example, acting intentionally increases the number of brain cells in the hippocampus, adds to the number of synapses, and enlarges its vault of knowledge and repertoire of mental and physical skills.

Summary: Discovering Your Life Purpose

Life's *purpose* is found in knowing, enjoying, and serving God. A meaningful life builds on that foundation through our *relationships* and *vocation*—expressing our talents and passions in our work and service.

Fortification refers to caring for the body and brain through wise lifestyle choices. Fortification is not synonymous with life's meaning. Instead, it helps equip us to do our best in all that we love and are called to do—spiritual life, relationships, and vocation.

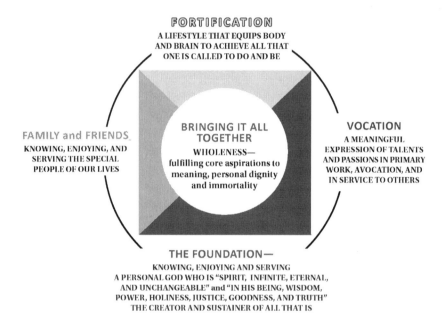

Vocation and Avocation

Your *vocation* is you; who you are; your enduring aptitudes, talents, gifts, passions, interests, personality and character. Ideally, your work is a consistent expression of your vocation; how God made you. An *avocation* is a complement to vocation. Both vocation and avocation describe who you are, but each may draw from a different set of talents and interests for a variety of reasons. One may not *want* to be engaged full time in an occupation, such as the talented artist who loves painting and drawing but doesn't want to do it forty hours a week. A person whose primary work is sedentary may take on a more physical avocational role such as a volunteer firefighter. One whose work is highly structured and repetitive may pursue creative expression through drama or art.

An avocation is distinct, often differing only in degree, from a hobby. A hobby is an activity I delight in, but it may not be as much a part of my personal identity as is my avocation. A hobby is an activity I enjoy doing. My avocation, like my primary vocation, is an important dimension of who I am.

HOW GOD MADE US

Generally, our vocational/avocational expressions are to be consistent with our talents, aptitudes, abilities, gifts, and passions—the way God made us. Sometimes God *equips* us with new abilities *at the time of need* to take on a new role or carry out a mission. It is also true that we may not yet be aware of some of our God-given aptitudes, so potential life choices will escape our consideration.

Meet Harry Lieberman with a renewed sense of purpose at age 79

At seventy-four, Harry Lieberman retired. At 79, he was somewhat bored with life but enjoyed playing chess at the Great Neck Golden Age Club in New York. On the day when his chess partner called in sick, a staff member pressed him to try his hand at painting in the art room. That experience struck a chord with Harry and motivated him to take a formal art course which launched a 26-year career and national recognition as a professional artist.

Harry Lieberman attributed his longevity (he lived to 106 years of age) to finding a sense of purpose in his art: "The art that I do is a part of Godness; it gives me a lift higher up." Harry's study of the Talmud and the Bible provided much of the subject matter in his watercolor and oil paintings.

Examples of God's calling in Scripture

Whom did God call to work alongside Moses when he said his burden was too heavy for him? It was "men of reputation" of maturity and judgment, empowered by the Holy Spirit.

- So the LORD said to Moses: "Gather to Me seventy men of the elders of Israel, whom you know to be the elders of the people and officers over them; I will take of the Spirit that is upon you and will put the same upon them; and they shall bear the burden of the people with you, that you may not bear it yourself alone." (Numbers 11:16-17)

- Whom did God call to accomplish the task of building the temple? They were laborers with strong backs: "Solomon selected 70,000 men to bear burdens, 80,000 to quarry stone in the mountains, and 3,600 to oversee them." There were also chosen gifted artists and craftsman, some of whom had to be recruited from Lebanon because there were none with the skills to cut timber from Judah or Jerusalem. (2 Chronicles 2:7-9)

- Whom did God call to write half of the New Testament? It was Paul, a most brilliant, disciplined and articulate scholar. Paul understood Greek thought and was trained in Judaism: "of the stock of Israel, of the tribe of Benjamin, a Hebrew of the Hebrews; concerning the law, a Pharisee." The intellectual capacity of Paul has been compared to some of the great philosophers preceding him.

- Whom did God call to write the detailed history recorded in the books of Luke and Acts? It was the physician, Luke. Luke's work, admired by Christian and non-Christian scholars alike, has often been put to the test by historians. It has withstood rigorous examination and deemed to be a reliable historical document.

Narrowing It Down

While God sometimes leads in dramatic ways, this is not the usual manner for which we are brought to an understanding of the work we are to train for and pursue. John Murray wrote,

> What path of life each individual is to follow in reference to this basic interest of life is to be determined by the proper gift which God has bestowed, and this is a key to the divine will and therefore to the divine call.

John Calvin recognized our tendency to grasp different things at once rather than realizing the benefit of recognizing the gifts God has given us:

> He (God) has appointed to all their particular duties

in all spheres of life. And that no one might rashly transgress the limits prescribed, He has styled such spheres of life, vocations, or callings. Every individual's line of life, therefore, is, as it were, a post assigned him by the Lord, that he might not wander about in uncertainty all his days.

KNOW YOURSELF - A KEY

You most likely won't know your calling unless you know yourself. If you are determining what career path to pursue, begin with your knowledge of yourself: your aptitudes, talents, personality, passions, and enduring interests.

Several "windows into your vocational soul" help discover what you can offer to the world of work and service, your: child heroes, personal aspirations and successes, most enjoyable experiences, and life purpose.

Childhood Heroes

Bill: I was seven years old. Joyce Taylor and I were playing together while arguing as to who would be Superman. She said she could be Superman, but I said, " You cannot be Superman because you are a girl." I strengthened my case by saying that I had a Superman suit. Joyce said, "Show me!" As she gazed at a suit comprised of blue-dyed long johns, a pair of red swimming trunks, a yellow belt with a gold buckle, a red cape, and the 'S' emblem for the chest crafted by my father, she said, "OK, you can be Superman. Put it on!" That ended the game. Superman was my hero, but no way was I going to be seen in public (except maybe for Halloween) in that getup.

My hero was Superman because he promoted justice, neutralized danger, and stood for the underdog. The themes that made up his story struck a chord. In adulthood, I chose the roles of teacher, co-strategist, counselor, and coach, working with people facing various life challenges. As a volunteer, my avocation was volunteer paramedic and fireman, allowing me to express values from my childhood.

Who are your heroes, and what qualities and values in you do they reveal? To what extent do they influence your life decisions, especially in vocation and work? Identify the careers or occupations best line up with your deeply rooted personal qualities.

Consider your heroes, the qualities you admire, and how those qualities correspond to careers or roles. What do you see in your heroes as a mirror of who you are in some way? How has your hero focus changed over the years, from childhood to the present?

SUCCESSES, ASPIRATIONS - TRIUMPHS GREAT AND SMALL

The Boxer

Outside my dressing room I heard the crowd as the last preliminary fight was ending. I felt the butterflies in my stomach. In a matter of minutes *I* would be standing in the ring in front of that crowd. Running off some nervous energy, I hit my gloves together and punched and jabbed the air. I was nine years old.

The crowd of fifteen to twenty neighborhood kids cheered as I stepped out of my dressing room—our basement—danced across the yard, and climbed between the ropes into the makeshift ring. Donned in a white robe, with gloves laced tight for battle, I was cast in the image of a pro.

Now seconds remained before the bell would signal the start of round one. Those tightly laced gloves thwarted a quick motion of my arms to shed the robe. They were much too big to fit through my sleeves. I felt the blood rush to my face as my energetic efforts to remove the robe served only to turn it inside out. Against the background of laughter, a grinning referee stepped forward to untie and remove my gloves to free my arms. No matter, dreams are often bigger than the obstacles they encounter. The fight came off as planned, and my dream of being a professional fighter lived on for still another year.

Children's aspirations, interests, and behaviors provide a window into the adults they are to become. What does the anecdote say about the one who constructs a boxing ring from his mother's clothesline and wooden props (without asking permission), organizes local kids to fight, recruits his best friend to compete with him in the main bout, and posts signs for the event across several neighborhoods to ensure a crowd? Unsurprisingly, the child became an adult who prefers to be his own boss, is goal-oriented and competitive, prefers to lead rather than being led, and is frustrated when he does not have the leverage or clout to make a significant difference in the world.

David – Connecting the Past to the Present

At age 16, David was asked to recall his earliest memory of personal success. After a long pause, he said it was the day he crossed the road, coming home from kindergarten. He said it was a success because it was a challenge and physical. "I did it by myself and then went home and shared it with Mom." (She firmly but gently told him to never again cross that highway again by himself.) Another success for David was wrestling. Again, it was physical and a challenge. He also enjoyed being on the mat with an opponent and being greeted afterward by his teammates and coach, win or lose.

What became David's career choice? It was emergency medicine, corresponding to what appealed to him when he crossed the highway—coming home from kindergarten by himself and participating in high school and college wrestling. It is a physical challenge involving independent effort and being part of a team. David built an extensive team practice integrating urgent care, family medicine, and preventive medicine. In keeping with his profile, David competed (and won) in the American Gladiators competition and was first in the physical competition in military officer training.

But this is about you: identify your successes as far as you can remember. No success is too far back, too small, or too big to consider. Each is a window into your lasting strengths, talents, or aptitudes able to contribute to success in a current or future job, occupation, or vocation. Today, they are a window into our vocational soul and help chart your life course.

Valued Experiences

Looking back, which of your life experiences have been most gratifying? Which of your successes do you associate with being the most enjoyable, valued, and rewarding? Passion exercised without corresponding talent leads to frustration; talent lacking in passion becomes wearisome.

The Executive

An executive is being groomed as the successor to the CEO in a corporation, a role for which he believed he was eminently qualified. As the move-up approached, he became anxious and somewhat distressed. Upon reflection, he recognized that his real passion was to work in a leadership role in which he could make a direct, measurable impact on human lives. Was it assisting those who are homeless? Hunger? Those addicted to drugs? Ministering to those with spiritual needs? Reaching out to men and women who are in prison? He had not yet narrowed his focus, but he knew it was time to move on. He walked away from the path he had been following, even though it was lucrative and prestigious. He knew he would be miserable if he stayed.

The Attorney

A young woman, a graduate at the top of her class in law school, earns a big salary with a large law firm and is positioned to become a partner. However, she is so consumed by her work that she has little time to invest her energy in other important areas of her life. She is unhappy and has decided to make some changes: resign from her position, open a business (with significantly reduced income), and invest in other areas of her life that she believes are highly valued and fulfilling.

In her shoes, would you make this life change?

Key Figures

Wes Stafford grew up in a missionary family. He lived with them in a remote village in Ivory Coast until he was old enough to attend boarding school. His experience there was horrendous, as described in his book, *Too Small to Ignore* (WaterBrook Press, 2007). Yet, these experiences led him to lead Compassion International and reach the lives of countless children who needed help.

Condoleezza Rice was the daughter of parents who determined their only child would not be limited by her gender or race, described in the book, *Condi*, The Condoleezza Rice Story (Zondervan, 2002) She rose to be Secretary of State under President Bush.

C. Everett Koop describes in his memoir, <u>Koop</u>, (Random House, 1991) of growing up in Brooklyn and how the doctors he knew as a young child contributed toward stirring his passion for medicine.

An Exercise in Daydreaming

Many of us spend half of our time wishing for things we could have if we didn't spend half of our time only wishing. (Stephanie Danielle Haff)

Suppose you awaken tomorrow with the freedom to enter any career, profession, or occupation you choose. Assume nothing is out of reach and you have all the knowledge, skill, and credentials to immediately to step into that position. What would you choose: *sales, medicine, education, art, athletics, homemaking, skilled labor, skilled crafts, music, drama, law enforcement, engineering, religion, finance, government, politics, astronomy, scientific research, the military, or business*? There is a myriad of other possibilities.

Choose what you would select as a long-term occupation. After making your selection, identify what appeals to you about that type of work. Why is it a good fit?

HOW SMART ARE YOU?

Chances are you underestimate yourself. Several decades ago Dr. Howard Gardner of Harvard developed a body of research regarding multiple-intelligences—a range of separate individual intelligences but coalescing in various day-to-day successes, activities, study, recreation, and work. He believes the I.Q. approach to intelligence is too narrow, limited, and misleading or in error—sometimes off by as many as 40 points.

Bill Revisits High School

Most of us have taken a group-administered IQ test like the one I completed in the 10th grade. Our scores were made available to teachers and counselors but not to the students.

About a dozen years after high school graduation, I revisited my high school and stopped to see Mr. Bishop, who had been my guidance counselor. One of his first questions was about what I was doing with my life. I spoke about a growing family, the work I had done, and that I was nearing completion of work for my Ph.D. He made a funny expression, raised his finger, and disappeared to the next room. I could hear a couple of file drawers open and close, and then he reappeared with a puzzled look. He held up a five by eight card with all my high school grades, my senior photo, my attendance record, and that previously unknown not-so-impressive 10th-grade IQ score, and said, "Why you are only average!"

As you reflect upon your past successes, jobs, roles, and activities you have enjoyed, determine how they relate to Dr. Gardner's multiple-intelligence categories. Especially consider how the various areas of talent come together for success in any venture. For example, a role in a movie or play as an actor requires a range of intelligences: bodily-kinesthetic, linguistic, intrapersonal, interpersonal, and possibly others. This concept of integrating intelligences applies to most jobs or roles.

Since the intelligences function together in various expressions, they are best developed in various combinations, not in isolation. For example, the multiple intelligences recruited in partner dancing include interpersonal, physical, musical, and artistic-spatial.

OVERCOMING THE CHALLENGES OF PERSONAL BARRIERS

Obstacles cannot crush me. Every obstacle yields to firm resolve. He who is fixed to a star does not change his mind. (Leonardo Da Vinci)

If some barrier stands in the way of your success, there are two paths available. Either you go around your limitations, focusing on your strengths, or you take on the challenge of overcoming weaknesses.

The story about John

It is helpful to make a distinction between internal and external barriers. External barriers are *obstacles* we encounter. Internal barriers are *encumbrances* that we find within ourselves. The following story represents both types.

Jack (not his real name) was a 16-year-old, eighth-grade student in a "school for exceptional children" diagnosed with learning disabilities. Students enrolled in the school would be awarded a certificate at the end of the 11th grade, but there would not be a senior year or an award of an actual diploma.

One day, his 8th-grade teacher, having witnessed Jack's academic ability (but also his lack of confidence), commented: "Jack, this is an excellent school. But I wonder why you are bussed so far to this school instead of attending the high school close to your home. Jack responded: "I will tell you why! I was in third grade. When the other students played outside during recess, I stayed at my desk to catch up. When the other students were playing outside, my teacher came back into the room and said, 'Jack, why don't you go out and play with the other kids? You are never going to be able to get this work anyway!' Mr. _____, right then and there, I quit! They sent me to this school when I got way behind in my work."

With Jack's approval, following a home visit with his parents (the father was a coal miner who had finished third grade, and his mother completed sixth grade), a meeting was held with the principal, teachers, and a guidance counselor in Jack's local high school. This paved the way for him to leave his current school almost immediately and enter the 10th grade in his neighborhood high school. At that school, he was surrounded by all the help he needed to succeed. Initially, Jack attended the new school with fear and trembling, but anxiety gave way to a growing confidence, and after three school years, he crossed the stage to receive his well-earned high school diploma. Beaming with an ear-to-ear smile, he walked up to the 8th grade teacher who initially created the bridge toward graduation and said, "If three years ago anyone ever told me I would be feeling *so good* by walking across a stage to receive a piece of paper, I would have laughed at them!"

Footnote: Jack's early barrier to learning was related to an eye problem. He succeed without ever it being corrected.

Keys to Maintaining *Perspective in Your Life*

Your paths of work and service are to line up with your capabilities. Know yourself well, and then choose a vocational or avocational path that lines up with your abilities, interests, and what you value most. It is surprising how many people overlook this basic principle. Most jobs, when considered individually, are rather limited in scope. They do not allow for a full expression of all our abilities and interests.

Your work or service is to be balanced with other important areas of life. Work within the context of a balanced life means that you have time for all the important things outside of work, including intimacy with the special people of your life, recreation, sleep, exercise, spiritual life, and for applying your talents in home and community.

Be discerning as you consider how you can best serve your community. When it comes to people's needs, the saying, *"the squeaky wheel gets the grease,"* tends to be true. Sometimes we are wise to gently push our way past the squeaky wheels of the world, the people who yell loudest, to reach out to those quiet persons whose cries for help can barely be heard. (A study of adolescent girls who had attempted suicide revealed that every single one *felt* a strong need to go to others for help in times of emotional stress, but only 4% of them were willing to go to others and *ask* for help.)

Respect every type of work and service. How easy it is in our culture to place one person or job above another. There are jobs with greater responsibility, visibility, and financial reward, but there are no *inferior* jobs. Each has an important place in our world. On what basis can we honestly say that one job is superior to another? Power and prestige don't necessarily result in satisfaction. In one research project, people were asked about the level of job satisfaction they experienced based on the work itself and the tasks they performed. It was not the lawyers, doctors, and corporate executives who reported the highest levels of job satisfaction, but rather the craftsmen and tradesmen: people who could see the fruit of their labors and who said they were happiest with their work.

When you have a worthwhile goal, take action, give it your best effort, and don't give up without a good reason for doing so. *Action is eloquence.* (William Shakespeare)

Are you retired? Stay off the shelf. Due to age, health, or other factors, folks sometimes assume that they have less to offer in the way of work or service. Our society's notion of retirement at age 65 is not based upon the potential of older adults but refers to an economically-based decision regarding retirement made in Germany in the mid-1800s. As long as we are breathing and conscious there is a place for us in the world, regardless of seeming limitations due to age or disability. Don't forget Harry Lieberman becoming an artist at the age of 79!

Dedicate your efforts to God, the One who formed you and gifted you. A statement of Jesus: "And whoever gives one of these little ones even a cup of cold water because he is a disciple, truly, I say to you, he will by no means lose his reward." (Matthew 10:42)

Be Realistic

Often, we hear an enthusiastic, well-meaning, very successful person such as Oprah, or a well-known sports figure, a teacher, or parent say, "If you give your very best, you can be anything you want to be; you can accomplish all that you aspire to." Sorry, that's not true!

- The best swimmers in the world, such as Michael Phelps who has earned 28 Olympic medals, have long torsos and short legs.

- The best distance runners have long, thin legs.

- Many top major league baseball players have 20/12 visual acuity, unusually quick reflexes, a superior ability to track moving objects, and superior in dynamic visual acuity – the ability to discriminate the fine details of a moving object. They say that Ted Williams of the Boston Red Sox could count the stitches on a fastball. He was also the last player to hit over .400 for an entire season. He batted 406 in 1941.

- David Epstein, senior editor at Sports Illustrated, and author of the book, *The Sports Gene* points out there are seventeen American men in history who have run under two hours and ten minutes in the marathon, and there were thirty-two Kalenjin men with long, thin legs who did it in a single year in October of 2011. The Kalenjin are a tribe in Kenya consisting of a population of less than the population of the city of Atlanta.

While it is true that you and I cannot accomplish all that we set out to do, most of us underestimate our capabilities. Consider Rashad Jennings, a junior in high school. Doctors said his asthma would prevent him from participating in sports. At 270 pounds, coaches said he was too fat and slow. His grade point average of 0.6 negated the possibility of college. No matter, he dreamed of becoming a running back and went out for the football team. As the fifth-string running back, he didn't expect much action, so he sat on the bench chomping M & M's and drinking Sprite during games. However, as Providence would have it, in the last game of the season, the four guys in his position ahead of him suffered injuries, and Rashad was sent into the game. No one predicted what was about to happen. He was handed the ball and ran thirty yards for a touchdown. In the fourteen plays he was in the game, he scored four touchdowns—two on offense and two on defense.

The following fall, Rashad attended a private school, repeating his junior year and completing his senior year. His brothers made it possible because they agreed to coach without receiving a salary, enabling Rashad could attend tuition free. Rashad's academic success, plus 56 touchdowns and 3,287 yards rushing earned him a football scholarship and a starting position as a freshman at the University of Pittsburgh.

But Pitt was not to be in his future. A severe family medical concern led him to return home near Lynchburg, Virginia. He eventually enrolled in Liberty University and continued in football, scoring forty-two touchdowns. In his professional career, he played for the Jacksonville Jaguars, Oakland Raiders, and the New York Giants, with the latter signing a fourteen-million-dollar contract in 2014.

Are you underestimating yourself? Are you willing to persevere even if it's hard work? Perhaps your learning curve for mastering a skill is long and slow; you may still have great potential. By being tenacious, you may rise to the top of your game. An accomplished Broadway star, who also teaches voice lessons, said she would take the student with the drive and discipline over the naturally gifted student who lacked the discipline any day.

An initial slow learning curve may be misleading. I recall a young athlete who seemed relatively slow to master the skills of wrestling. One of his coaches, feeling frustrated and impatient with him during a team practice, knocked on his forehead several times, asking, "Are you in there?" I bet the coach was surprised to learn that the athlete later won a state championship, was a two-time All-American in college, and established himself as a world-class athlete, winning the Gold in the 2000 Pan American Championships and later finishing 10th in the world in the World Freestyle Wrestling Championships.

Would You Hire This Guy?

A young man, an exceptional student-athlete, was within weeks of graduation from college. To get a jumpstart on the job market he managed to schedule an interview with the president of the top finance and insurance company in the area. Arriving a few minutes early he introduced himself to the receptionist and made himself at home in the waiting area. His relaxed demeanor was in keeping with the T-shirt, shorts, and flip-flops he wore. When he met with the company president, he seemed quite at ease as he leaned back in his chair with his legs stretched out. Then he made a choking gesture by grasping the front of his neck while turning his head side-to-side and asked, "Do you have to wear a *tie* for this job?"

He was applying for a sales position. Intuitively, the president formed a positive opinion of the man and offered him a challenge: "Take this stack of forms to be filled out by prospective customers and return them to me." Within days he was back with every form completed. He was hired and eventually became the company's top salesperson. He was the top producer for many, many years. I never did hear if he ever wore a tie to work.

It is so easy to miss the God-given potential in ourselves and in others. As the receptionist was stuck by his demeanor and his mode of dress she laughed to herself and said, "That young man is 'dead in the water.' We won't see him again!"

BALANCING WORK AND RECREATIONAL ACTIVITY

There is an old saying, "All work and no play makes Jack a dull boy." It is also true "all play and no work" will eventually leave you and me with a sense of emptiness. The fancy word for it is ennui (pronounced ahn-wee), meaning a feeling of weariness, dissatisfaction, discontent or boredom. There needs to be a balance of work and recreative expression if we are to fulfill God's calling and to be equipped to serve effectively. Life activities either build us up or tear us down; they either restore, vitalize, invigorate, energize—or they dissipate. Dissipation is the squandering of personal energy and resources; it is the antithesis of recreative pursuits.

The concept of re-creativity, restorative rest, is built right into creation. We read in the book of Genesis that God created the heavens, the earth and all living things in six days. On the seventh day, He rested. The primary focus of the Sabbath concept is rest—rest for the land, one year in seven; rest for man and beast, one day in seven:

> Six years you shall sow your land and gather in its produce, but the seventh year you shall let it rest and lie fallow, that the poor of your people may eat; and what they leave, the beasts of the field may eat. In like manner you shall do with your vineyard and your olive grove. Six days you shall do your work, and on the seventh day, you shall rest, that your ox and your donkey may rest, and the son of your female servant and the stranger may be refreshed. (Exodus 23:10-12)

An essential guide for assessing the validity of any religion, worldview, or belief is to ask, "Does my thinking truly work in the real world? Can I live consistently with it?" In chapter three, we asked a practical question: as I live out the teachings of a religion, does it promote good or ill for me, for those around me, and for the world?

Taking one day in seven to rest from our work makes sense, but the concept goes beyond one day in seven. Current research confirms that we do well to rest daily, during our workday, and at the end of each workday. Many of us run on a daily high dose of adrenaline, which, over time, will cause damage to the body and brain. Studies have shown even a twenty-minute, restful break during the workday will break the cycle of adrenaline and an excess buildup of cortisol, enabling us to avoid consequent injury to our bodily organs and significant disease.

You are the best person to discern if you need more refueling time. Look at the total time spent in restful or recreative, edifying activities for the week. Now ask yourself how you are feeling. Are you relaxed? Are you renewed? If not, perhaps you may physically or emotionally require more time spent on these recreational activities.

And then there are vacations—those longer times of rest each year we are supposed to find restorative. It doesn't make sense a vacation should be a stressful, whirlwind experience that takes several days (or longer) to recover from. Sensible, thoughtful planning is in order when scheduling a vacation.

Some employers have a policy of allowing their staff to take an extended period, six months to a year, for a sabbatical leave. Many school districts, for example, allow a staff member to take six months to a year off, at half salary, after 6 or 7 years of service. A person who takes advantage of the policy may have much more to give when they return to the formal workplace.

The dictionary defines the word sensible as "a course of action chosen in accordance with wisdom or prudence; likely to be of benefit." Are we sensible by taking the time we need for recreation; daily, weekly, or yearly?

Woody Allen says, "Most of the time, I don't have much fun; the rest of the time I don't have any fun at all." If Woody's statement describes you, you may be long overdue for a change.

IN SUMMARY

Self-knowledge is key to choosing or reaffirming your life's work. Take the time to view yourself through the windows described above: Your heroes and personal aspirations throughout childhood; successes great and small, from your earliest memories to the present; enjoyable, valued, and rewarding experiences; and where you have found life meaning or purpose.

An additional valuable source is what others say about you. Consider interviewing trusted family members, friends, and coworkers who have had an opportunity to observe you in various settings and under diverse circumstances. What are the passions, interests, strengths, weaknesses, successes, and failures that have been evident to them? Ask each person for evidence-based responses, not flattery or words of affirmation.

Watch out for the dream killers. People in your circle might be threatened if you change. They may like things the way they are. The fear monster can get in the way of success. Fear is a tap on the shoulder to get our attention. It is not to be the final arbiter of what we are doing. Analyze the facts, and make intelligent, informed decisions, but if all systems are on the "go," even if you are shaking and trembling, move ahead!

May we be able to say when we leave this earth that we have used what God has given us to make a positive difference in the world and the lives of the people God brings our way.

CHAPTER 5

DEVELOPING YOUR EMOTIONAL SELF

Amy was a single mother for several years, raising four daughters between the ages of 8 and 15. As is often the case, working, caring for children, and running a home can be taxing. One evening, Amy entered the door, and the girls were watching TV. She was tired and went straight into the kitchen. The dirty dinner dishes were still on the table, and the kitchen was messy. Amy lost it. She stormed into the TV room and not so quietly ordered them to clean up. As she went to her bedroom, the girls scurried.

When Amy returned, it was very quiet. She apologized for losing her temper. She explained that she had worked all day and felt unappreciated when coming home to a messy kitchen. The girls listened and understood, promising to do better. Then one of them respectfully and kindly said, "But how do you think we feel when we haven't seen you all day and before you even say hello, you yell at us." Amy got the message and committed to taking a different approach.

Positive and negative emotions are a central part of our lives and can catch us by surprise. For example, imagine how we feel when we're in jeopardy of losing a job: anxious and maybe even angry; when we are in a troubling relationship: hurt, fearful, insecure; when we've completed a degree: excited and proud. Our feelings influence how we operate as we engage with the world. Emotions make up a critical piece of communication. In a sense, they are a language of their own. Have you ever looked at someone across a room and perceived they were feeling sad or anxious before even conversing with that person? As integral as our emotions are to our daily lives, we want to manage them well.

How well, or not so well, we express our emotions plays a significant role in the quality of our relationships with God and the special people in our lives; our physical health—e.g., unresolved guilt and anger are powerful forces behind clinical depression and our ability to invest ourselves in exercise and engage in re-creative activities.

Growing up, we learn how to manage and express emotion. In some families and cultures, the outward expression of emotion is discouraged, and talking about harmful and painful experiences is always unwelcome. For example, many soldiers who served in WWII are characterized by not sharing the ongoing feelings associated with their encounters. Some families don't do emotions at all—the rule is to suppress and deny. In other families, the full expression of emotion is encouraged, even to the point of yelling.

A woman in her thirties talked about her family of origin and mentioned that she was in her thirties before she realized you didn't have to manage every disagreement with intense anger. That was contrary to the behaviors she had learned from two parents who constantly yelled at each other and the children, sometimes even throwing things at one another.

Of course, we learn from sources other than the family: the church, school, peers, neighbors, extended family members, culture, and society. Can we free ourselves from negative influences? Wouldn't it be great if, when we reach adulthood, we could do a comprehensive debriefing for our lives? We could evaluate what we have learned, correct and redirect what is counterproductive, and then move forward having learned to express and manage our emotions and lives well.

The good news is that it is never too late. The truth is it is a lifelong journey to become experts at what we might call emotional literacy. We can begin by exploring our past, how we got to where we are now—getting in touch with our emotions and feelings, what are their sources, understanding the influence they have over us, how to process and let go of counterproductive emotions, and finally how to express them well. (We may also benefit from outside resources that can counsel us on managing life's significant areas or psychological/medical issues that hinder us from moving forward positively.)

In this chapter, we are looking at how to be emotionally fit so that we are equipped to relate well to God and others, function in all the spheres we're engaged in, and enjoy all God has called us to and has for us.

Being emotionally well encompasses a healthy interaction of our thoughts, feelings, and behavior. It isn't very easy. Feelings spring from our behavior and thoughts. (E.g., I feel guilty when I act contrary to what I think is right.) It is also true that behavior and thoughts result from our feelings (e.g., I love my child, so I think and act to protect them from danger.) In another situation, I flee when experiencing fear in the face of danger, despite believing I should stay and fight.) As our best selves, we are in touch with our feelings, and we express those feelings appropriately, but our feelings do not have the last word as the ultimate determiner of our actions. The foundation for our feelings and behavior is what we think—what we believe. And what we believe should be judged by what is true.

It is appropriately choosing what to do rather than allowing our emotions to control us. Think of the time you were shaking in your boots before your commitment to stepping on stage as a public speaker, the school exam you were anxious about, or the butterflies before your part in a performance or an athletic event.

Bill: I recall the dry mouth, high anxiety, feeling physically weak, and the fear of failing in front of my peers and a panel of judges before a test in Taekwondo. I thought, "I can't do this; I will look like an idiot. Let me out of here!" But I went ahead, to fail or succeed, saying, "I must." To my surprise, things went well. My fear was an inaccurate predictor of my performance. And quitting was not an option.

Beliefs, Emotions, and Behavior

- Our beliefs provide the foundation for our feelings and behavior. Our thoughts and beliefs give birth to our emotions and feelings.

- Our emotions and feelings reveal our thoughts.

- Our thoughts, and our emotions/feelings, consciously or unconsciously, work together and find expression in our moment-by-moment choices and actions.

- Our thoughts and behavior are a window into our soul. "As in water face reflects face, so the heart of man reflects the man." (Proverbs 27:19)

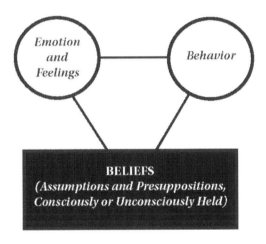

EMOTIONAL WELL-BEING

You are emotionally healthy when:

- You have the *inner* capacity to exercise your personal freedom spiritually, relationally, sexually, vocationally, recreationally, and physically. *It takes all of life to make a life.*

- Overall, you characteristically choose to behave in a manner that promotes your well-being and the good of others.

- You have an accurate perception of yourself, your life and your world.

- Your choices are in accord with what is true, and what is right. Your feelings and the expression of your emotions fit the reality of yourself, your world, and your circumstances.

- You are the same person in all contexts, not putting on a facade in front of others.

The freedom enjoyed by an emotionally healthy person stands in contrast with the limitations which accompany:

- *Neurosis*, in which a person is entangled in a web of repetitive, self-defeating thoughts or behaviors

- *Psychosis*, having difficulty in discerning what is real and what is not real

- *Addiction,* being in the throes of being dependent on a destructive substance such as drugs, alcohol, or tobacco

- *Self-defeating habit*, being held captive by patterns that do not promote your well-being

THE HEART OF THE MATTER

Our life experiences shape and mold us. They teach us who we are, how to view the world, and relate to others. To the degree that what we learn is healthy and accurate, these beliefs positively impact us. Some experiences, however, have the potential to distort our beliefs and have a negative impact on our thoughts and feelings. From time to time, it is wise to take an inventory of our heart-held beliefs, identify their sources, assess their impact on our lives for good or ill, and challenge those ideas that do not pass the test of truth. There is an old saying, "Time heals all wounds." By itself, time will not heal either a severe physical wound or a deep emotional wound. Left unattended, unresolved issues from the past siphon off our energy and hijack our emotions, attitudes, thoughts, and behaviors in the present.

What is your emotional climate? What is characteristic of your emotional world and underlying beliefs? How did you arrive at this emotional place? How do you manage and express your emotions?

Assess yourself in the light of the feelings described on the next page. Consider the steps you need to take for growth or change:

- *I feel a sense of personal power or clout or leverage when it comes to impacting and shaping my life, my world, and the people around me.* Am I on top of my world, or is the world on top of me?

- *I am feeling free, unfettered.* Are there elements or dimensions of my life that are stifled or hindered, standing in the way of what I believe I am called to be and to do in life?

- *I am feeling at peace; I am experiencing contentment.* Do I experience inner peace, or am I continually wrestling with, or suppressing anxiety, fear, guilt, discontent, shame, deep grief, disillusionment, hurt, or anger?

- *I feel a sense of personal satisfaction.* Not that I have arrived, but do I feel pretty good about my life and who I am?

- *I am optimistic, overall.* Characteristically, do I hold a confident, positive outlook, or am I wading through pessimism?

- *I feel connected with my world and the special people of my life.* Do I enjoy intimate relationships and adequate meaningful time with my most important people?

- *I feel full, fulfilled in life.* Am I working through a significant loss? Are there areas (spaces) in my life that are highly valued, but are empty or partially empty?

In this chapter, we encourage you to identify and challenge negative patterns. Let's define more precisely what we mean here. We are looking at two factors that impact our emotions: core beliefs and closure. (Some behaviors and emotional issues are rooted in spiritual, psychological, or physical issues best served by a corresponding professional—pastoral counselor, therapist, or physician.)

The messages we embrace form our core beliefs. What do you believe on the deepest level of your being?

- What do I believe, and why?
- What do I know *for sure*?

- What or who is my authority—my source of truth?
- How can I know right from wrong?
- How can I separate out what is true from what is not true?
- How do my beliefs line up with the teaching of my source(s) of authority—for example, how do the beliefs and assertions of the authors of this book line up with the teaching of Scripture?
- What is the connection between what I believe, and my day-to-day decisions and lifestyle?

How much of your view of self is derived from what others have said of you and how they have responded to you? Who are your mirrors? Are they plate glass backed with silver, conveying an accurate image, or of the amusement park variety that can distort the truth and precious worth of who you are? What do you believe on the deepest level of your being? Core beliefs will find expression in your day-to-day emotions and behavior. False, misguided beliefs will sabotage your life. Heart-level beliefs direct our day-to-day choices. What is the source of my beliefs? Do they correspond to who I am and the real world? How do my beliefs shape my life? Scripture encourages us to sift through and embrace the evidence set before us. The physician, Luke, the author of the New Testament books of Luke and Acts, invites us to do so with eyewitness testimony and reliable historical documentation:

> Inasmuch as many have undertaken to compile a narrative of the things that have been accomplished among us, just as those who from the beginning were eyewitnesses and ministers of the word have delivered them to us, it seemed good to me also, having followed all things closely for some time past, to write an orderly account for you, most excellent Theophilus, that you may have certainty concerning the things you have been taught. (Luke 1:1-4)

And Peter, another New Testament author, invites us to take our brain through the door of faith—not a blind leap of faith, but a belief based on the available evidence. Peter's directive is for believers being "prepared to make a defense to anyone who asks you for a reason for the hope that is in you, yet do it with gentleness and respect." (1 Peter 3:15)

IDENTIFYING OUR INTERNAL TRUTHS

Daryl

The forces shaping our thinking begin at birth (if not before) and have a lasting impact on our lives. In a meeting with first-grader Daryl, an elementary counselor stood ten large rubber dolls in a line on a table. He told Daryl, "The first guy is the smartest kid in your school. The second guy is smarter than all except the first. The last in the line is not as smart as the others. All the students in the school are smarter than him." The counselor then asked Daryl which doll represented him. Without hesitation, Daryl pointed to the last in the line, the least intelligent.

Daryl was bright, but at the end of the last school year, his twin sister had been promoted to second grade while he was held back. It had nothing to do with intelligence; instead, he had some catching up to do developmentally—especially in his reading.

The counselor then changed the script. He told Daryl the first rubber doll guy in the line was the toughest kid in school; he could beat up all others in a fight. The second guy can beat up everyone except the first guy. The guy at the end, everyone can beat him up. The counselor again asked Daryl which best represented him. Daryl, with a glance at the floor, conveyed an expression of modesty, jabbing his finger toward the first guy, the toughest. His choice was backed by a reputation. A few days earlier, he had chased a big 5th grader down the street, following him right into the middle of his living room. The boy's mother intervened to break up the fight and rescue her son.

How could we help Daryl see himself differently and recognize his ability when he believed he was stupid? Words alone would never accomplish the goal. A better route is to bring him to question and challenge his false impression of himself. In effect, he begins to consider that even though he feels stupid, maybe he is not. As soon as he is willing to question his false assumptions about himself, he becomes open to new evidence. That new evidence, over time, becomes persuasive. Ultimately, it overturns and replaces the old belief. For example, in the old mindset, getting an "A" on a test was a fluke; now, the "A" becomes evidence that maybe Daryl is smart.

Patricia

Patricia was playing with her friends on the school playground. The teacher noticed that whenever Patricia spoke with another, she took hold of the child's arm and pulled her toward herself. The teacher quietly and gently asked, "I notice that you always take hold of a friend's arm when you speak. Why do you do that? Patricia said without hesitation, "If I don't do that, no one will listen to me!"

The teacher tried to learn more about the child and her family. She discovered Patricia had many siblings, including a newborn, and had faded into the woodwork. She had gotten lost in the family crowd. The family welcomed the intervention by the teacher on Patricia's behalf, and things took a positive turn for her.

Consider: What did your growing-up years teach you about yourself, men, women, God, and the world? Scripture says, "As a man thinks in his heart, so is he." (Proverbs 23:7). What we believe and how we think will, indeed, determine the course of our lives, whether we will be at peace or anxious, happy or miserable; experience the sweet smell of success or the bitter taste of repeated failure; sometimes even whether we live or die. Our beliefs provide the blueprint for the life we're going to build.

A few examples of the power of belief

The men and women below believed they were at the mercy of external circumstances rather than having control over what happened to them. Belief shaped their destiny.

1. **A tribal member** has broken a taboo. The "witch doctor" points a bone at the man, a gesture that brings the curse of death. His family begins digging his grave and preparing for his funeral. In two days, he is dead.

    The outcome explained: *The tribal member,* knowing that he was "cursed," believed he was going to die. If the same witch doctor pointed the bone at you or me, we would simply shake our heads and laugh.

2. **A homeless man** climbs into a train car and pulls the door shut, realizing too late he has locked himself in the refrigerator car. Hours later, when a member of the crew opens the door, he finds the man's lifeless body and sees a message scratched onto the wall: "Help me, I'm freezing to death."

    The outcome explained: *The homeless man* as it turns out, had locked himself in a refrigerator car and it was not turned on – the temperature was not low enough to cause death by hypothermia. He believed he was freezing to death and he died.

3. **A group of patients** are released from a mental hospital,

but within a short span of time, a high percentage of them relapse and are again hospitalized. Patients in a second group were released but tmost of them did not relapse.

The outcome explained: Each patient who relapsed was told they were doing well and being released because of their treatments. At the same time, those in the second group of patients with similar diagnostic profiles were told they were being released because of the steps they had taken to better their lives, not because of medication or medical treatments. The second group with the low relapse rate had experienced a sense of strength, hope, and freedom, believing they had a say in their lives.

4. **A prisoner of war** in Viet Nam, in relatively good health and known for his resilience, suddenly begins to deteriorate and dies.

    The outcome explained: the *prisoner of war* had come to firmly believe he would never be free and went into a steep decline with the loss of all hope.

5. **Sixteen of seventeen elderly women** die after moving to a home for the aged—8 within 4 weeks and 8 more within ten weeks.

    The outcome explained: *Sixteen women* died believing they no longer have the freedom to shape their lives, and the home for the aged symbolized there was nothing worth living for.

King David

David is a well-known Biblical figure. The power of belief is evident in every aspect of his life. In the Old Testament, King David was called a man after God's own heart. He was a beloved King of Israel. We read of his adventures with intrigue and excitement, anticipating each venture's conclusion. His personality shines throughout the Psalms. His genuine vulnerability in relating to Saul, Jonathan, Nathan, and others is revealed in other Biblical texts. At times, David's choices cost him dearly. It is painful to read on as these storylines unfold.

Although David is first mentioned in the Book of Ruth, we begin to get to know him in the Book of I Samuel. Samuel, God's anointed prophet, is sent to Bethlehem to see a man named Jesse. God has informed Samuel He has chosen a son of Jesse to be King over Israel.

When Samuel first arrived, he invited Jesse and his sons to the sacrifice he would present to God. Samuel is impressed by the seven young men who stand before him, but none are the anointed one. God says "no" to each.

> And Jesse made seven of his sons pass before Samuel. And Samuel said to Jesse, "The LORD has not chosen these." Then Samuel said to Jesse, "Are all your sons here?" And he said, "There remains yet the youngest, but behold, he is keeping the sheep." And Samuel said to Jesse, "Send and get him, for we will not sit down till he comes here." And he sent and brought him in. Now he was ruddy and had beautiful eyes and was handsome. And the LORD said, "Arise, anoint him, for this is he." (1 Samuel 16:10-12)

The Spirit of the Lord came upon David from that day forward, but he was not immediately put on the throne. In fact, he returned to tending sheep.

Meanwhile, back on the home front, King Saul is not doing well. The Spirit of the Lord left him, and an evil spirit was tormenting him. He is desperate for comfort and hears about David's soothing musical abilities. Samuel sends a messenger to Jesse and requests David be sent to court to play for him. Whenever Saul was distressed, he called for David to play for him. Saul is so pleased with David that he makes him an armor bearer. Now enters the champion of the Philistines, Goliath:

> He stood and shouted to the ranks of Israel, "Why have you come out to draw up for battle? Am I not a Philistine, and are you not servants of Saul? Choose a man for yourselves, and let him come down to me. If he is able to fight with me and kill me, then we will be your servants. But if I prevail against him and kill him, then you shall be our servants and serve us." And the Philistine said, "I defy the ranks of Israel this day. Give me a man, that we may fight together." When Saul and all Israel heard these words of the Philistine, they were dismayed and greatly afraid. (1 Samuel 17:8-11)

David's seven brothers are engaged in the war, and Goliath has taken a stand against the Israelite soldiers for forty days. David, still going back and forth from the court to tending sheep, is now sent by his father to take grain, cheese, and bread to his brothers, who are knee-deep in the battle. It is interesting to read in I Samuel 17:28

how David's oldest brother responds to seeing his young sibling:

> When Eliab, David's oldest brother, heard him speaking with the men, he burned with anger at him and asked, "Why have you come down here? And with whom did you leave those few sheep in the wilderness? I know how conceited you are and how wicked your heart is; you came down only to watch the battle."

This is not the warm, welcoming response we expect from David's brother. As we read further, we see how Saul turns on David. He torments and, on multiple occasions, attempts to kill him. He spends years in the land of the Philistines, running from Saul. Amid the betrayal by many others, David found a trusted friend in Jonathan. He loved Jonathan more than a brother.

If we put ourselves in David's place, how did his experiences shape his beliefs, and how did his beliefs shape his choices, such as his affair with Bathsheba, the murder of Uriah, and his unwillingness to deal appropriately with his sons, Amnon and Absalom.

What about you?

- What negative beliefs were forged by my past?
- How will my beliefs shape my future?
- How does my relationship with God and my beliefs about Him inform my choices?
- What are my beliefs about myself? For example, how much say do I have in determining my future?

CLOSURE

A lack of closure refers to an ongoing emotional burden of past experiences that negatively impact our current life. Primary negative emotions often associated with a need for closure include guilt, anger, grief, and fear. We may or may not be consciously aware of their presence and influence on our moment-by-moment feelings, thoughts, and behaviors.

Achieving closure is often used to describe bringing an issue to a state of completion, resolution, or finality. For our purposes, closure is defined as understanding the impact of an incident in our lives that caused pain or harm and processing the emotions around that event to the degree that we can constructively manage the emotions surrounding the event.

Closure does not mean that we never recall the past or that it no longer stirs up any emotion at some point. We know several families who have lost a child or more than one child: in one case, two brothers; in another, a son, daughter, and grandson. The parents of these children will always have feelings and never stop thinking of these loved ones. We remember the special people in our lives who are no longer here. While emotions from past experiences may never disappear entirely when we have closure, they lose power and no longer control us. Bill lost his younger brother, Bob, when he was only in his mid-forties. When Bill asked his Dad if he often thought of Bob, he said with some emotion, "Yes, every day."

As you will see in the following examples, closure is not just about loss.

Leroy

Leroy and his wife have a counseling appointment with the pastor, but Leroy seems in no hurry. He sat down in the kitchen with a plateful of food. His wife is concerned they will be late for their appointment and asks Leroy to hurry. Leroy jumps up from the table and throws the plate against the wall. The plate shatters, and the food splatters. Leroy storms out of the room.

It was no surprise that when they reached their appointment, the incident became the focus of the discussion. Along the way, the pastor asked Leroy if his wife's message to hurry along reminded him of anything in his past. Leroy thought for a moment and then described his mother, who had a way of always showing up, being ever-present. "If I went to the basement, she was there; if I went to the porch, she would be there. Not only was she always correcting me, always making adjustments to something about me, being critical, but I couldn't escape her constant scrutiny."

Leroy's outburst in the kitchen was fueled by previous experiences with his mother: being constantly under his mother's watchful and critical eye. He perceived his wife as an extension of his mother's behavior, viewing him as inadequate. The primary experience of inadequacy and feeling indignant found expression in the secondary emotion of anger.

Soldiers on a Secret Mission

A soldier awakened to find his younger companion absent from their tent. He found him outside, some distance away, shaking and sweating. The veteran asked if he was having nightmares stemming from past war experiences. He shook his head yes and asked if they would ever go away. The seasoned veteran smiled and gently responded, *"No, but you learn to make them your friends."*

Jeff

Jeff is highly regarded by friends and coworkers. To see him, you would assume all was well. But no one goes unscathed by destructive childhood experiences. Jeff grew up with an alcoholic father. When he was young, Dad would come home drunk and wreak havoc in the home, breaking things and verbally abusing his wife. He often approached Jeff with a hostile posture and threatening words. Jeff prepared to defend himself, hiding an easily accessible baseball bat under his bed. Not lacking in courage, he was ready for the drunken, angry man who might invade his room. Wrestling through the painful memories of Dad and the hurt and anger he felt toward Mom for not walking away and protecting him, he sought the help of a counselor. Eventually, he realized it was time to put the bat down. The young boy who was rightfully hurt and angry was healing, and Jeff, the man, adopted constructive ways to deal with past adversity.

Craig

Craig also had a painfully difficult relationship with his father. The criticism and belittling were constant. His father conveyed Craig was a loser who would never amount to anything. His experiences in school reflected his father's words. He was neither a good student nor did he have the confidence to engage in athletics and other skilled activities. He did not gain acceptance among his peer group. What ultimately saved Craig was relationships with Christian leaders who invested in him, provided guidance, and genuinely conveyed they were with and for him. As he moved into adulthood, he was able to embrace his strengths to experience what any observer would call success.

What About You?

Are you held captive by a lack of closure? An overreaction to a situation with intense emotion and reactive behavior may indicate that unresolved issues from the past are impacting your life in the present. A lack of closure *may* reveal itself through:

- any acting out behaviors

- unexplained anxiety or phobias
- depression
- difficulty sleeping
- unwillingness to take risks
- use of food, alcohol, drugs to manage emotional pain
- a pattern of poor, destructive relationship choices
- impulsive spending
- exaggerated feelings of grief over minor losses
- great feelings of guilt over seeming minor infractions
- negative eating patterns
- unexplainable chronic physical symptoms
- weight gain
- an unusually strong need to be in control
- habitual self-defeating patterns of behavior

Suppose our emotions are hindering us somehow, either by being suppressed or being expressed openly in negative behaviors. In that case, it is timely to identify and work through any unresolved, emotionally charged experiences from our past. Strong feelings are bound to rise to the surface when choosing to walk the path of healing. As we revisit painful memories and experiences, these feelings can be overwhelming. As F. Scott Fitzgerald put it, "In a real dark night of the soul, it is always three o'clock in the morning, day after day." (The Crack-Up, 1945).

It is essential to create a robust support system. The process is a journey and requires patience and perseverance. It is hard work. Proverbs 18:4 gives us an indication of the burden: "The human spirit can endure in sickness, but a crushed spirit who can bear?" God promises that He will walk with us. "A bruised reed he will not break, and a smoldering wick he will not snuff out. In faithfulness, he will bring forth justice." (Isaiah 42:3)

There is a broad range of possibilities regarding unresolved emotions and feelings, such as anger, guilt, shame, fear, anxiety, grief, hurt, injustice, inadequacy, and disillusionment. We'll look at some of these in more depth.

ANGER

John and Clara were in their eighties. John was severely disabled with rheumatoid arthritis. He asked for assistance as he struggled to rise from his chair. As he stood, he groaned, showing strong feelings of pain and frustration. In one instance, John was again struggling to stand. Clara, usually soft-spoken, shouted, "That's why you are crippled! You're angry, and keep it all inside!"

Indeed, he was angry. He had harbored searing anger and resentment with the death of his young son many decades earlier. Possibly Clara's statement was true. His anger may have been a factor in his disease. It certainly could have exacerbated his condition if it was not a root cause.

Unresolved anger can lead to a variety of signs and symptoms. It can:

- be a "pain in the neck" and cause recurring headaches
- alter the appetite
- bring on fatigue
- compromise the immune system
- contribute to hyperactivity of the digestive tract, ulcers, high blood pressure, skin blotches and bumps
- precipitate a heart attack
- express itself in the form of depression (common in men)
- disrupt relationships and inhibit intimacy
- erupt in a flash of temper
- enslave a person in a vicious cycle of self-defeating behaviors
- be irritable and liberal in giving out criticism without being able to receive criticism

Anger finds it hard to forgive another. An angry teenager was once asked why she would not forgive her parents. Her answer "Because then I would have to stop punishing them!"

Holding to anger can victimize us further. A man whose wife was killed in a fire blamed the firefighters who fought the fire and filed a lawsuit against them. There was a lengthy investigation by a neutral party, and no evidence of neglect was found. Although tragic, the loss of his wife was an accident. The fire company was not culpable. The grieving widower angrily refused to accept the decision and vowed to pursue it further, even if it took the rest of his life.

We are commanded to rid ourselves of the poison anger creates: "But now you must also rid yourselves of all such things as these: anger, rage, malice, slander, and filthy language from your lips." (Colossians 3:8; NIV)

We don't want anger to consume us. The first step toward

managing anger is to identify the primary emotion or feelings underneath the anger—anger is often a secondary emotion, masking the root cause. Are you angry? Identify your underlying feelings. Is it hurt, fear, sadness, injustice, grief, frustration?

After identifying your primary emotion and its source, plan the next step you can take to resolve the issue. For example, is there one with whom you need to reconcile? Sometimes, we may feel an "either-or" situation in which we blast another or suppress our feelings and walk away. There is a third way. It is not to confront but to communicate with dignity, strength, and gentleness. Yet, be prepared for the various responses from the other person you may elicit. You cannot control the other person but can do your part. It may be helpful to conduct a role play with a friend you can trust, in which your friend acts out the possible responses you may face.

Have you identified unresolved anger in the face of injustice? Biblically based principles provide a framework for managing anger in the face of evil and injustice (often at the root of anger). The framework includes four truths:

First, anger is an appropriate response to evil, but even justifiable anger can be wrongly managed, becoming ugly and destructive. "Do not take revenge, my dear friends, but leave room for God's wrath, for it is written: 'It is mine to avenge; I will repay,' says the Lord." *(*Romans 12:29)

Second, God is absolutely sovereign. He is in control and nothing is by chance. While God is not the author of evil, even the evil acts of men and women He limits and directs to His glory and to the building up of His people. Romans 8:28 tells us God causes all things to work together for good to those who love Him.

Third, God is just and will work justice in accord with His own timetable. When injustice comes into our lives, it is under the sovereignty of God. Scripture says the Son of God appeared to destroy the devil's work (I John 3:8). We are commissioned to continue the work of Jesus in destroying the works of the devil, overturning the consequences of sin in the world. It may not be worked out even in our lifetime, but God's promise of justice will not be broken. Having used up each God-appointed means for dealing with injustice and still not being satisfied, we give the matter over to God, who judges with complete fairness.

Fourth, God is gracious and merciful: "while we were yet enemies of Christ, He died for us." He who has promised to work justice has satisfied the demands of justice on our behalf. Consider what Christ has done and wants to do for us. This should soften our hearts to forgive others.

GUILT AND SHAME

Psychiatrist Karl Menninger reminds us of sin's great problem in his book Whatever Became of Sin? He states that the great human problem is GUILT. He chides clergy who are timid and compromising in calling sin. Guilt and its companion, shame, are to be reckoned with.

Guilt is the experience of falling short of an ethical standard; shame is the sense of morally falling short as a person. Shame is experienced most intensely when our guilt falls under the gaze of another, especially the gaze of God. Think about Adam and Eve covering their nakedness and shame after they violated God's command. Recall Nietzsche's statement, "Man killed God because he couldn't stand to have God looking on his ugliest side. Man must cease to feel guilty." Without God, true guilt disappears, and without guilt, shame has no place. For the Christian, there is awareness of moral absolutes, real guilt, and shame, and in Christ, the way of redemption, forgiveness, and new life.

A seven-year-old Patrick was regularly stealing coins from his grandmother's dresser drawer. He felt guilty. One day, he played with his friend Jimmy on the stone-paved street in front of his home. His parents sat watching from the front porch. As Patrick bent down to pick up a stick, his stolen coins fell from his shirt pocket and bounced on the stones. As his mother sternly ordered, "Pat, come up here," his sense of shame overshadowed his guilt. Conscience brings awareness of transgression and guilt; being guilty while under the gaze of others brings a sense of shame.

Some folks grow up in homes where a parent, a grandparent, or another significant figure is an expert at eliciting guilt. Failing to honor and love one's parents is guilt-worthy. However, failing to meet certain expectations of the parent does not make one guilty or a terrible son or daughter. In addition to dealing with the inappropriate experience of guilt from the past, we want to see the ongoing manipulative patterns and not continue to buy into false guilt.

George

George was grown and married, but his mother continued to find various ways to elicit guilt in him. There were two instances when George failed to meet his mother's expectations, and she subsequently developed chest pains, called 911, and was taken to an emergency room. George had been working on understanding her posture toward him throughout his childhood and adulthood. He began catching on to her manipulation and took a stand. George and his wife, Cynthia, planned to travel to Europe for a vacation. Anticipating another emergency room visit by his mother, George announced their plans:

> George: Mom, I am stopping by to say "good-bye."
>
> Mom: What do you mean? It sounds rather final!
>
> George: Yes, Cynthia and I are heading off to Europe for a week's vacation. I know you have had heart problems, and if something would happen when we are away, I want to make sure I had said good-bye.
>
> Mom: She was silent, but her facial expression shouted, "How could you, my son, abandon me? You know I have a bad heart!"

George and Cynthia completed their journey to Europe. Mom was safe and sound when they returned and had made no emergency trips to the hospital. She experienced no chest pains or other heart symptoms while they were gone. George and Cynthia's choice to travel was wise, liberating, and guilt-free.

Guilty, or not?

The first step toward resolving guilt is establishing whether we are truly guilty. The accusations of others and our conscience can lie to us. We need to first differentiate between what is true guilt and what is false guilt. True guilt occurs when we have failed to do what we ought to, such as not stepping up to help a person being treated unjustly, turning away from one in need, or mistreating others through prejudice, lying, cheating, or stealing. Actual guilt is when we violate the laws that God has established to protect a person's dignity.

Some situations are not so black and white. John Murray addresses this truth in his book *Principles of Conduct,* saying, "At the point of divergence, the difference between right and wrong, between truth and the lie, is not a chasm but a razor's edge." He refers to the narrative of God telling Samuel to go to Jesse and choose a king from among one of his sons:

> And Samuel said, "How can I go? If Saul hears it, he will kill me." And the LORD said, "Take a heifer with you and say, 'I have come to sacrifice to the LORD.'

> And invite Jesse to the sacrifice, and I will show you what you shall do. And you shall anoint for me him whom I declare to you." Samuel did what the LORD commanded and came to Bethlehem. The elders of the city came to meet him trembling and said, "Do you come peaceably?" And he said, "Peaceably; I have come to sacrifice to the LORD. Consecrate yourselves, and come with me to the sacrifice." And he consecrated Jesse and his sons and invited them to the sacrifice. (1 Samuel 16:4-5)

Did Samuel lie when the elders greeted him as he came to Bethlehem? He did not lie, nor was he obliged to reveal his primary mission. Sometimes, we prayerfully wrestle long and hard with issues, poring over relevant Scripture and seeking the wisdom of others before discerning God's way, the right way to go.

Yogi Berra said, "When you come to a fork in the road, take it." All humor aside, many forks in the road demand a choice. In the face of an apparent dilemma, there is a right and better way to go. Our conscience is a vital guide; if we remember it is not infallible. It can be ill-informed, excusing us when we've done wrong and accusing us when we've done right. The conscience is not the final word. God's word is our authority and is to inform our conscience. When the conscience falsely accuses or excuses, we are to challenge it from the teaching of Scripture. Dr. Francis Schaeffer remarked, "If your conscience falsely accuses you, you should kick it across the street!"

The same rule applies when others falsely accuse us of wrongdoing. Test it by the Scriptures. Udo Middleman's previously quoted statement is worth repeating, "We have a propensity for adding to the Word of God and binding one another's consciences with what we believe to be right." Our consciences are to be informed by God's word. Once we identify that we have committed an offense and are guilty, we need to take care of business by acknowledging and confessing our sins. Holding on to our sin will destroy us from the inside out. David describes what he felt before confession:

> When I kept silent, my bones wasted away through my groaning all day long. For day and night, your hand was heavy upon me; my strength was sapped as in the heat of summer. Then I acknowledged my sin to you and did not cover my iniquity. I said, 'I will confess my transgressions to the Lord, and you forgave the guilt of my sin.' (Psalm 32:3-5)

Beyond Confession

Confessing our sin is the doorway to emotional freedom, removing the barrier between us and fellowship with God. The general rule is to ask forgiveness from those we have offended. Pray for wisdom regarding to whom we should confess and the proper timing. An untimely confession may bring a sense of relief while placing a crushing burden on another. At the same time, we need to be aware if we are rationalizing away our obligation to confess to another.

Dealing with sin does not end with acknowledgment and confession. We are instructed to make things right. There are circumstances when restitution is necessary. In the Old Testament, restitution goes beyond what has been taken from another.

> The LORD spoke to Moses, saying, "If anyone sins and commits a breach of faith against the LORD by deceiving his neighbor in a matter of deposit or security, or through robbery, or if he has oppressed his neighbor or has found something lost and lied about it, swearing falsely—in any of all the things that people do and sin thereby—if he has sinned and has realized his guilt and will restore what he took by robbery or what he got by oppression or the deposit that was committed to him or the lost thing that he found or anything about which he has sworn falsely, he shall restore it in full and shall add a fifth to it, and give it to him to whom it belongs on the day he realizes his guilt." (Leviticus 6:1-5)

The spirit of the law carries over into the New Testament in the teachings of Jesus. Sometimes, restitution is costly and can be a hard step to take. Consider seeking wise counsel as to how to proceed. However, stopping short of taking this step will prohibit us from reaching a place of full strength and freedom. It is an area where we are to trust God as well.

King David's Example

When Nathan confronted David about his adultery with Bathsheba and the murder of her husband, David confessed, saying, "I have sinned against the LORD." In Psalm 51, he prays,

> Have mercy on me, O God, according to your steadfast love; according to your abundant mercy blot out my transgressions. Wash me thoroughly from my iniquity, and cleanse me from my sin! For I know my transgressions, and my sin is ever before me. Against

you, you only, have I sinned and done what is evil in your sight, so that you may be justified in your words and blameless in your judgment. (Psalms 51:1-4)

David continues his plea: "Create in me a pure heart, O God, and renew a steadfast spirit within me." (Psalm 51:10). Like David, we are to own up to our sin in repentance. What is to follow repentance is found in Christ's words to the woman caught in adultery. The religious leaders brought the woman to him, saying that Moses said such a person should be stoned:

> Now in the Law Moses commanded us to stone such women. So what do you say?" ... And as they continued to ask him, he stood up and said to them, "Let him who is without sin among you be the first to throw a stone at her." And once more he bent down and wrote on the ground. But when they heard it, they went away one by one, beginning with the older ones, and Jesus was left alone with the woman standing before him. Jesus stood up and said to her, "Woman, where are they? Has no one condemned you?" She said, "No one, Lord." And Jesus said, "Neither do I condemn you; go, and from now on sin no more." (John 8:5-11)

God Forgives Completely: Forgiven Sin is Sin No Longer Remembered

When Christ announced that Peter would betray Him, He also said, "But I have prayed for you, Simon, that your faith may not fail. And when you have turned back, strengthen your brothers." (Luke 22:32) The message to Peter was that despite his failure, Christ would be with him and bring Him back. Christ loved Peter, would not forsake him, and had a plan for his life. Can our offense be any greater than Peter's?

After we confess our sins, we are not to continue to accuse ourselves or bathe ourselves in guilt and shame. In embracing God's forgiveness, forgive yourself. "Come now, let us reason together, says the LORD: though your sins are like scarlet, they shall be as white as snow; though they are red like crimson, they shall become like wool. (Isaiah 1:18)

God's forgiving ways may be difficult for us to grasp, not only because of the magnitude of sin when measured against the Holiness of God but because it is often so foreign to what we experience in day-to-day relationships. Typical is the attitude, "I can forgive, but I can't forget." God's promises are the opposite: "For I will forgive their iniquity, and their sin I will remember no more" (Jeremiah 31:34)

A Child's Perspective

I entered the living room and saw my son, Matthew, age 4, pinching himself. I asked him the obvious question: "Matthew! Why are you pinching yourself? "I hurt David," was his reply. We talked. I shared God's clear steps to complete forgiveness as we sat together. I said, "And when Jesus has forgiven you, you are not to punish yourself." He responded with a big smile while turning his head side-to-side, saying, "Daddy, no one ever told me that in my whole life!" He had heard the message many times, but there was a particular context this time.

God's loving commitment is sacrificial: Christ said, "Greater love has no one than this, that he lay down his life for his friends. You are my friends if you do what I command." (John 15:3). His relationship with us is permanent. "I give them eternal life, and they shall never perish; no one can snatch them out of my hand. My Father, who has given them to me, is greater than all; no one can snatch them out of my Father's hand. I and the Father are one." (John 10:28-30). There is nothing we can do to increase or decrease God's love for us; it is based on who He is and what He has done on our behalf. It is not based on our performance.

FEAR AND ANXIETY

The phrase "fear not" is repeated often in the Bible. Fear is a common experience for all of us and is a theme addressed from Genesis to Revelation. We see fear enter our world immediately after Adam sinned. In Genesis 3:9-10 (NIV): "But the Lord God called to the man, "Where are you?" He answered, "I heard you in the garden, and I was afraid because I was naked, so I hid." God knows our natural tendency to be afraid, and the truth is living in a fallen world where sin abounds can be a scary thing. Bad things do happen.

In Matthew chapter three, we find John the Baptist imprisoned, the prospect of death looming over him. He began to struggle with doubt. He sent a messenger to ask Jesus if he was, in fact, the One who was to come. Like John, we are prone to doubt in threatening or overwhelming circumstances.

To experience fear in the face of a threat is understandable. Fear can be a good thing, awakening us to danger. The key is to manage fear wisely, drawing from God's strength. As we stated earlier, fear is a tap on the shoulder to get our attention, but the experience of fear itself should not direct our steps as the final arbiter of our decisions.

Rules have exceptions. In teaching personal safety and self-defense, we have instructed students to be aware of their surroundings and also be aware of a "gut feeling" that suggests danger lies ahead. If a scene elicits fear and you do not have sufficient evidence to alleviate your fear, then listen to your gut. You may be responding to subtle cues that you can't quite articulate.

If we receive a phone call informing us that a family member or friend has been taken to the emergency room, we would naturally feel anxious and fearful. What gets us into trouble is anxiety or fear controlling a portion of our lives, limiting us from embracing what God has for us and pursuing what He has called us to do. The goal is to be able to respond appropriately rather than walking around feeling anxious and afraid. Anxiety can present itself in a variety of ways, such as:

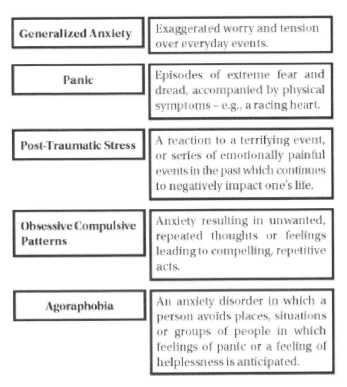

Generalized Anxiety	Exaggerated worry and tension over everyday events.
Panic	Episodes of extreme fear and dread, accompanied by physical symptoms – e.g., a racing heart.
Post-Traumatic Stress	A reaction to a terrifying event, or series of emotionally painful events in the past which continues to negatively impact one's life.
Obsessive Compulsive Patterns	Anxiety resulting in unwanted, repeated thoughts or feelings leading to compelling, repetitive acts.
Agoraphobia	An anxiety disorder in which a person avoids places, situations or groups of people in which feelings of panic or a feeling of helplessness is anticipated.

General symptoms of anxiety are:

- Panic, fear, and uneasiness
- Sleep problems
- Not being able to stay calm and still
- Cold, sweaty, numb or tingling hands or feet
- Shortness of breath
- Heart palpitations
- Dry mouth
- Nausea
- Tense muscles
- Dizziness

Paul gives us guidance as to our proper response to anxiety:

> Do not be anxious about anything, but in every situation, by prayer and petition, with thanksgiving, present your requests to God. And the peace of God, which transcends all understanding, will guard your hearts and your minds in Christ Jesus. (Philippians 4:6-7)

Managing Fear and Anxiety

God is compassionate and understands our fear. We see him being a God of encouragement in his instructions to Joshua:

> No man shall be able to stand before you all the days of your life. Just as I was with Moses, so I will be with you. I will not leave you or forsake you. Be strong and courageous, for you shall cause this people to inherit the land that I swore to their fathers to give them. Only be strong and very courageous, being careful to do according to all the law that Moses my servant commanded you. Do not turn from it to the right hand or to the left, that you may have good success wherever you go. (Joshua 1:5-7)

The goal is to manage fear and anxiety so that while we know they exist, they no longer control us, our decisions, or our behavior. Fear becomes nothing more than a tap on our shoulder to get our attention.

There is no magic switch to flip and turn our emotions and feelings off, but the following can be extremely helpful in managing our feelings while we are working through any unresolved issues that may be at their root:

- ☐ Exercise – a great way to 'walk-off' anxiety

- ☐ Healthy eating – stay away from foods that can contribute toward feeling hyper

- ☐ Relationships – allow others to be a listening ear and talk through what your feeling

- ☐ Prayer and meditation – in addition to staying connected with God, God wants to be part of the process with you and his Word is replete with encouragement and guidance

- ☐ Professional Counselor - It may be helpful to work with a professional who can provide insight, techniques, and medication to work successfully work through fear and anxiety.

In reviewing the list above, which of these tools do you consider to be the best tools for managing fear and anxiety?

GRIEF

Amy: One afternoon, my daughter, who was in elementary school, walked into the kitchen and asked if she could talk to me. She rarely initiated such discussions. Her usual response to how her day went was "fine," and that was that. I knew she was troubled. We went outside where her sisters wouldn't bother us. We sat on the front steps, and I asked her what was happening. She said she didn't know what she would ever do if I died. She was getting close to the age when my mother died, so I shared with her what it was like for me. We talked about who was there and who helped me. We named the people in her life who would be there for her. In the end, I asked her if she felt better. She said she did but added, "But I don't think I'd ever stop crying." A loss is hard, even if it's only thinking about it.

Loss is an integral part of our fallen, imperfect world. In a sense, you could say overcoming loss is an ongoing theme for all of us. When we hear the word loss, most of us immediately think of death but dealing with loss takes on many forms: loss of a loved one, a job, finances, health, youth, a social structure or culture, a cherished possession, security, identity, a title, our innocence, or significance.

Take a woman in her sixties who was attending group therapy. The group was instructed to choose various pictures cut out from magazines and arrange them in a collage. No other guidelines were given. Her collection was filled with attractive scenes—beautiful locations, young women, and flattering clothes. Yet, she had a look of sadness on her face. It seemed contrary to the images she had placed in front of her. When asked to describe her feelings, she said the collage represented her life in bygone days when she traveled to faraway places, wore lovely outfits and jewelry, and had her youth. She grieved the loss of a bygone era, which was never to return.

We can also experience loss over an aspiration never achieved. A man in his thirties lost his father unexpectedly. They had not been close, and his father had never said he loved or was proud of him. When his father died, the young man grieved not only the death but also the father he desired and would never have. There was no longer any hope of the relationship he had dreamed of. It is normal to experience grief when we experience loss, and the grieving process can take time.

If you uncover memories leading to a grieving experience, be aware that healing may include various stages that can shift back and forth: denial, anger, bargaining, depression, and acceptance.

Mishandling of loss and grief can lead to an increased risk for psychological concerns, relational disruptions, and health risks. Behaviors one might notice:

- Failure to move on with life
- Blaming self or others
- Internalizing feelings resulting in depression and even worse, suicidal ideation
- Isolation
- Acting out in a destructive, hurtful manner toward self or others
- Resorting to the use of drugs and/or alcohol to escape
- Distorted thinking

Managing Grief

- Grief is a powerful emotion and how we process grief can vary from one person to the next.

- Some individuals show their emotions outwardly and cry with friends and loved ones. Sharing our journey with the appropriate people God brings our way can go a long way in helping us to work through our feelings. There was a mother who toured the country sharing about the loss of her child in a senseless drive-by shooting. It was painful to hear. One interviewer asked how she was able to keep going over and over these disturbing events. Her response, *"Because every time I tell it the hurt is a little less."*

- Expressing feelings through journaling or poetry can be consoling.

- Engaging in physical activities can be an avenue for processing grief; activities such as hiking, sailing, running, and working with our hands.

- A young man who lost his wife spent a year remodeling the house until he completed every project he and his wife had dreamed of doing. The outlet gave him a constructive path for expressing the tremendous need to invest himself in meaningful activity until he was able to express himself verbally.

- Christian author and speaker, Elizabeth Elliot (1926 – 2015), was asked how she got through her grief after her husband was martyred. She said, "I just did the next thing." That was an important part of her answer, but the fullness of her response included her faith in God, trusting Him as he sustained her during her indescribable pain. Elisabeth believed that suffering is never for nothing—even when one cannot make sense of their loss.

- Never be a Lone Ranger during times of loss.

About Forgiveness

Sometimes, a lack of closure is mixed with grief because we have not forgiven the person we have lost. Achieving closure can be a long and arduous process. If someone has caused injury, there are many issues, including hurt and injustice.

Forgiveness begins with a posture of humility and brokenness. Pray God will soften your heart and help you move toward and trust Him. Regardless of your feelings, seek to be obedient to his calling in your life. (Remember Joseph and his brothers).

Forgiving others may include bringing the offense out into the open:

> If your brother sins against you, go and show him his fault, between the two of you. If he listens to you, you have won your brother over. But if he will not listen, take one or two others along, so that every matter may be established by the testimony of two or three witnesses." (Matthew 18:15-16)

If the offender will not take responsibility by acknowledging wrongdoing, it is not the end of the matter. We are still to get our hearts right with God. We want to be where we are ready to forgive those who commit offenses against us. Whenever they are ready to ask for forgiveness, we can extend it. If the offense against us is never acknowledged, and we have fulfilled all God calls us to do, we are to take the offense to the Lord and leave it in his hands to complete either in this life or the next.

Forgiveness does not mean we will, or should, reinstate those to the place they once held when they have done wrong. There are consequences to sin, and there is a difference between forgiveness and trust. If a person has stolen from us, we may not soon again choose to allow the person to be in our home or our employment. When trust is broken, persons often lose the privileges they once had, even though forgiven.

Unwillingness to forgive has everlasting consequences: "But if you do not forgive men their sins, your Father will not forgive your sins." (Matthew 6:15) God calls us to forgive: "But if your brother sins, rebuke him, and if he repents, forgive him. If he sins against you seven times in a day, and comes back to you and says, 'I repent,' forgive him." (Luke 17:3-4)

What About You?

None of us can accurately claim that we have arrived. We can get to a place where we can say, with gratitude, that we feel good about where we are and our path. How are you doing?

- Do you have a vision for your emotional well-being and plan to take you there?

- Are you ready to take the next steps to implement that plan?

THE POWER OF CHOICE

There are two parallel Biblical truths stated in Scripture. God is absolutely sovereign, and we make real choices that impact our lives and our world. There is no logical contradiction between the two and no need to diminish one side of the equation to the elevation of the other. They are both already affirmed as true throughout God's teaching. God has a plan for our lives, and we are responsible for making healthy choices to live out that plan. We reside in a culture that resists the sovereignty of God. For some, there is no need for God at all. For others, God exists but does not have much say or authority over our lives.

A well-known, often-quoted line illustrates the diminishing of God's sovereignty while elevating the power of our choices. It is William Ernest Henley's poem, Invictus (Latin, "unconquered"): "I am the master of my fate: I am the captain of my soul."

Henley, it is said, was an avowed atheist. He attributed his unconquerable soul to "whatever gods may be." But it appears the gods he refers to have left him to defend for himself. And defend and fight he did. He was a man of courage and inner strength, which carried him through the storm of an impoverished childhood. He experienced much pain and suffering from tubercular arthritis of the bone, taking one leg and threatening to take the other. The intervention of a "determined, persevering surgeon" spared the leg. Despite the surgeon's efforts, tuberculosis eventually took Henley's life at 53. His life experiences taught him much, influencing significant core beliefs about himself and the world, but unfortunately, no recognition of the One who created all that is.

Life, for all of us, will have some difficult chapters. Here is some encouragement from folks who have overcome.

SOME INSPIRING STORIES
BEING A VICTIM DOESN'T MEAN STAYING A VICTIM

Jane

Consider a woman we will call Jane. Jane was not doing well. She was depressed, experiencing intestinal problems, and missing work. These behaviors were not typical of her. She decided to see a counselor. Jane shared that her boss was an angry, intimidating woman. Jane was wilting under constant scrutiny and criticism and felt powerless to change how her boss treated her. She became a victim of the oppressive environment the woman's demeaning patterns created. While it was clear her boss was the trigger, Jane's response was extreme.

Jane began to explore the details of her home life growing up, where children were to be seen and not heard. She was not permitted to challenge authority; if she dared to rock the boat, she was a 'bad' girl and punished by being sent to her room for long periods.

It comes as no surprise that Jane, as an adult, felt tremendously inadequate when she was in situations where she had to speak up for herself. She had embraced learned helplessness. As Jane worked through her hurt and rejection, she began to differentiate between Jane, the child, and Jane, the adult. Slowly, she began to set boundaries with her boss and was eventually able to stand in a place of strength.

Jane was a victim of destructive childhood experiences and carried a victim mentality into adulthood: a target, helpless, inadequate, and not in control. Victimization can teach people these things, but we will not flourish if we're unwilling to shed this identity and replace it with the truth.

The following anecdote was first aired on the nationwide radio program "Focus on the Family" many years ago and is a beautiful picture of shedding the label of being a victim.

Anna

Anna grew up in a small town. Her family had little money, but it didn't matter to her. She didn't care about going on to college. More than anything else, desired to be a wife and mom. She was enjoying her high school years, looking forward to her graduation and the future that awaited her and her boyfriend. While driving home from an after-school activity one evening, the weather took a turn for the worst. A bad storm hit, and as she descended a narrow, hilly road, a truck skidded across her lane and hit her head-on. She was paralyzed from the waist down. Her dreams were crushed, as was her spirit. After months of hospitalization, surgery, and rehab, her mother took her home. She felt what it was like to be a helpless child. Initially, her mom had to help do almost everything.

The family fell into an acceptable routine, but she was understandably depressed and agitated, never dressing but only wearing pajamas. One morning after breakfast, her mom entered her room and put Anna's jeans on the bottom of the bed. Anna asked her mother what she was doing. Her mom said it was time for her to get out of her pajamas and put on her jeans. Anna screamed angrily at her mother: "Why are you doing this? I can't do anything! What's wrong with you?" Her mother left the room.

After an hour of ranting and raving, Anna stared at the jeans. Slowly, she reached down and was able to grab them. She tugged, pulled, and cried, and then cried some more. It continued for a long time, but Anna finally got her jeans on.

Then Anna shouted for joy. Then she heard her mother crying from the other room, where she had been waiting the entire time. Mom's tears were not those of despair over the difficult recent months but a celebration of a much-needed victory in her daughter's life. This insightful and courageous mother knew her daughter could not live the rest of her life as a victim. She had reached a crossroads and made the right choice. Anna was the first physically challenged individual to attend a local college. She completed her degree and later married and had children.

Frank

In his twenties, Frank went on permanent disability. He was hospitalized many times over the years, at least twice a year in recent years. He believed he would never be able to work for a living. Frank made a firm decision to redirect his life. He began an exercise program and, over several months, began feeling better and looking better, and was pleased by his improved physical fitness. Eventually, he dared to dip his big toe into the pool of the frightening world of work. He initially took on a volunteer role, securing a part-time job working for the owner of a print shop. He did so well that the owner offered him a permanent, paid position. Frank thanked her but said he wanted to explore other volunteer work options before settling into a venture long-term. His next step was to volunteer at an assisted living and nursing center. He found that he was making a difference in some lives and was greatly appreciated by the residents and the staff.

Frank became emboldened. The man who thought he would never be able to work for a living decided to offer his services for a fee to older adults in the wider community. He established a proprietorship, created a logo, and designed and distributed attractive brochures. Before long, he was getting requests to offer his helping hand. His business thrived, and he was flourishing. He waved the fee if a person in need could not afford to pay for his services. He continued to see his psychiatrist for a while, who affirmed him and complimented him on the rewarding paths he had chosen. The need for hospitalizations ceased.

Frank continued adding building blocks to his life. He continued with his exercise program, taking notice of his improved aerobic fitness and strength. He changed his diet, lost weight, stepped away from one unhealthy relationship, and began investing in two new friendships. He found his work rewarding, appreciating the frequent expressions of gratitude from those he served. Even his view and understanding of God changed, and there was renewal in his spiritual life.

The many years that have gone by are a testimony to Frank's courage and an affirmation of the decision to change his life. He became a different man, with a quality of life that far surpassed anything he had previously imagined.

Frank's (and your) internal gyroscope

Frank's life is an excellent testimony to the power of taking small steps forward, tackling one life area at a time. It is like having an *internal gyroscope*. A gyroscope consists of a wheel spinning within a frame.

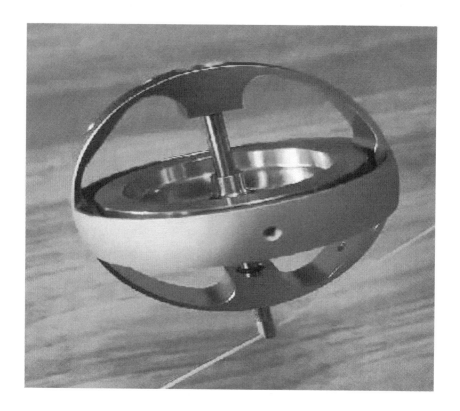

When the wheel is spinning at great speed, it provides stability for systems ranging from ships' navigational equipment to vehicles for space travel. The principle of the gyroscope is central to what God built into the universe—it is called angular momentum. The spinning of planets, solar systems, stars (including our sun), and galaxies contribute to the stability of our universe. The rapid rotation, for example, contributes to the Earth not collapsing into the sun.

Engaging one's internal gyroscope allows one to move forward with spiritual strength and emotional and physical stability in the face of many obstacles and challenges. Like Frank, when we are on track, investing in life's essentials—spiritual, social, vocational, recreative, physical, emotional—provides stability parallel to that provided by the angular momentum of a gyroscope. It allows us to take on and overcome the internal and external challenges we encounter with greater strength and confidence.

If we are running on empty in one or more of life's major areas, we are less able to take on the more difficult things that come our way. Frank's bold steps undoubtedly gave him the stability and strength necessary to be freed from all that had held him back for many years.

We are to take responsibility and initiative to move forward, but we are not alone. God gives us the power, guidance, people, and other resources to succeed. Sometimes, we can only explain an outcome due to God's intervention, bringing us to our discussion of Joseph in the Old Testament.

Joseph

You may recall that Joseph was the favorite of his father, Jacob, and his brothers were jealous. So jealous that they conspired to kill him. One of his brothers had compassion, and instead, Joseph was thrown into a pit and sold to some passing traders. They, in turn, sold him to Potiphar, an Egyptian captain of the guard in the service of Pharaoh.

Meanwhile, Joseph's brothers reported to their father that animals had killed him. The chapters of Joseph's life unfold. He moves from a favored position in Potiphar's household, only to be falsely accused of attempted rape by Potiphar's wife. He spends more than two years in prison and then rises to a position of power—second in command only to Pharaoh himself.

One day, Joseph had some surprise guests. His brothers were in Egypt searching for food because of a great famine. Egypt, thanks to Joseph, was doing all right. When the brothers were first escorted into Joseph's presence, they did not recognize him. Eventually, Joseph revealed who he was:

> Joseph could no longer control himself before all his attendants, and he cried out, "Have everyone leave my presence!" So there was no one with Joseph when he made himself known to his brothers. And he wept so loudly that the Egyptians heard him, and Pharaoh's household heard about it.
>
> Joseph said to his brothers, "I am Joseph! Is my father still living?" But his brothers were not able to answer him, because they were terrified at his presence.
>
> Then Joseph said to his brothers, "Come close to me." When they had done so, he said, "I am your brother Joseph, the one you sold into Egypt! And

now, do not be distressed and do not be angry with yourselves for selling me here, because it was to save lives that God sent me ahead of you. For two years now there has been famine in the land, and for the next five years, there will be no plowing and reaping. But God sent me ahead of you to preserve for you a remnant on earth and to save your lives by a great deliverance. (Genesis 45:1-7; NIV)

As for you, you meant evil against me, but God meant it for good, to bring it about that many people should be kept alive, as they are today. (Genesis 50:20)

CONCLUSION

God is a God of timing. As we seek his direction in our lives, we can be at peace if we trust His agenda. Although we may want to hurry things up, God may have other plans. We can pray for God to reveal what we need to explore as He equips us to move forward. He leads and directs our steps: "Listen, my son, accept what I say, and the years of your life will be many. I guide you in the way of wisdom and lead you along straight paths. When you walk, your steps will not be hampered; when you run, you will not stumble." (Proverbs 4:10-12; NIV). Continue to have hope. God promises to be with us in our suffering and pain: "Weeping may stay for the night, but rejoicing comes in the morning." (Psalm 30:5) And, "In this world, you will have trouble. But take heart! I have overcome the world." (John 16:33)

God is Truth: He would have us believe the truth about ourselves, others, the world and universe, and himself. Core beliefs are deeply rooted beliefs from which we interpret our experiences. Our beliefs inform and shape our choices.

In Philippians Paul states:

Finally, brethren, whatever things are true, whatever things are noble, whatever things are just, whatever things are pure, whatever things are lovely, whatever things are of good report, if there is any virtue and if there is anything praiseworthy—meditate on these things. (Philippians 4:8)

A word of caution is needed here if you are in a controlling and abusive relationship. As you begin to heal, the abuser may be threatened by your growth and increase their efforts to control or manipulate. Stay on track and surround yourself with caring, trustworthy folks. A psychologist shared some words of wisdom for dealing with negative feedback. His message was when criticized, listen carefully, stand alongside your critic, and, looking at yourself, consider what is accurately based on evidence and what is not. Usually, your best defense is no defense; learn and apply what is helpful from the criticism.

Cast aside what you know to be false. Be informed by reliable sources you can count on and talk to yourself accordingly. The well-known physician-turned-pastor, Dr. Martyn Lloyd-Jones, reminds us King David talked to himself rather than listening to himself. The following is from Lloyd-Jones' book entitled Spiritual Depression:

> I say that we must talk to ourselves instead of allowing "ourselves" to talk to us! Do you realize what that means? I suggest that the main trouble in this whole matter of spiritual depression in a sense is this, that we allow our self to talk to us instead of talking to our self. Have you realized that most of your unhappiness in life is due to the fact that you are listening to yourself instead of talking to yourself?
>
> The main art in the matter of spiritual living is to know how to handle yourself. You have to take yourself in hand, you have to address yourself, preach to yourself, question yourself. And then you must go on to remind yourself of God, Who God is, and what God is and What God has done, and what God has pledged Himself to do.

If you are unaware of unresolved closure issues and are not experiencing any barriers in living out your life or reaching your goals, leave well enough alone. As the saying goes, don't fix it if it's not broken. We can pray God brings to light anything from our past if He needs us to come to terms with an issue. A thought by Reinhold Niebuhr:

> Living one day at a time,
> Enjoying one moment at a time,
> Accepting hardship as the pathway to peace.
> Taking, as He did, this sinful world as it is, not as I would have it.
> Trusting that He will make all things right if I surrender to His will.

CHAPTER 6
FORTIFY AND ENRICH YOUR BODY

YOUR AMAZING BODY

Reflect on King David's exclamation:

> For you formed my inward parts; you knitted me together in my mother's womb. I praise you, for I am fearfully and wonderfully made. Wonderful are your works; my soul knows it very well. My frame was not hidden from you, when I was being made in secret, intricately woven in the depths of the earth. (Psa 139:13-15)

Imagine what he would say today, given the wonders of the human body and brain continuously being explored by modern science. Try to wrap your brain around what is described in the pages that follow:

The Cell - Consider the amazing 37.2 trillion cells in the human body, all buzzing with activity. Each cell is a tiny universe. It includes an array of mechanisms for building and tearing down "roads" traversed by strange-looking, self-propelled vehicles—motor proteins—designed to transport waste out of the cell.

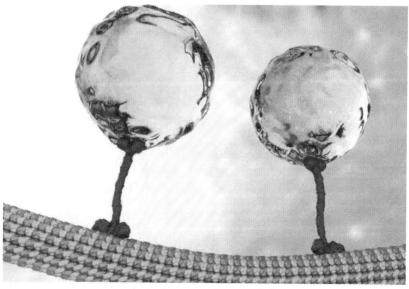

A motor protein at work

The cell contains special mechanisms for bringing oxygen, glucose, and other nutrients into the cell. The mind-boggling one billion chemical reactions per second are indispensable for the cell's life and are made possible by the 2,000 enzymes produced within.

Red Blood Cells - Red blood cells are the smallest cells in the body, with a diameter of about one-eighth to one-tenth of the width of the average human hair. There are about twenty-five trillion red blood cells in the body. The life of these cells is about three to four months, so they must be replaced at the rate of three million per second! Each red blood cell contains about 250 million hemoglobin molecules, capable of transporting one billion life-giving oxygen molecules.

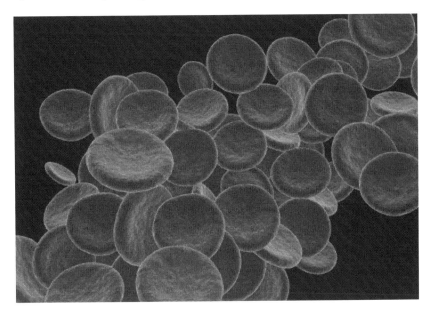

Red blood cells

Response to Injury - How we are protected from bleeding to death from a simple wound is another amazing process designed by our Creator. You may not care to put this process to memory, but reading through will give you an appreciation for its complexity. Platelets, fragments of large cells produced in both bone marrow and the lungs, are attracted to damaged tissue; a slice, cut or puncture wound. The platelets adhere to damaged blood vessels, forming a platelet plug. The plug releases chemicals resulting in the narrowing (vasoconstriction) of the blood vessels. The platelets also release other chemicals to combine with plasma to produce thromboplastin. Thromboplastin acts as an enzyme to activate prothrombin, converting it to the active form, thrombin. In turn, thrombin works to convert the soluble protein fibrinogen into the insoluble protein fibrin. Fibrin molecules join in a mesh around the wound, trapping blood cells to form a blood clot.

There is more. Platelets cause retraction of the clot, pulling the fibrin strands to bring the edges of the wound closer together. Because the plasma proteins prothrombin and fibrinogen are neutralized by enzymes immediately after they form, the clotting is limited to the area of the wound. Otherwise, clotting would spread throughout the body, forming a deadly giant clot. God thought of everything, didn't He?

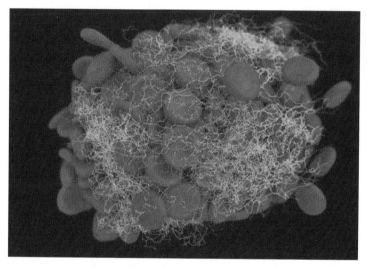

[Luk Cox] © 123RF.com
The clotting process

The Spine - Consider how God, the Greatest Engineer, ensured the structural stability of the spine, and why it doesn't usually buckle when subjected to heavy loads.

Because of the connecting structures of the muscles which function like guy wires, the spinal column maintains its structural integrity when subjected to strong compressive forces. In his book entitled, *Low Back Disorders* (pp. 113-114), renowned back expert Dr. Stuart McGill, Professor of Spine Biomechanics at the University of Waterloo, presents an interesting illustration:

> Suppose a fishing rod is placed upright and vertical with the butt on the ground. If the rod were to have a small load placed in its tip, perhaps a pound or two, it would soon bend and buckle. Now suppose that the same rod has guy wires attached at different levels along its length and that those wires are also

attached to the ground in a circular pattern. Each wire is pulled to the same tension (this is critical). Now if the tip of the rod is loaded as before, the rod can sustain the compressive forces successfully. If you reduce the tension of just one of the wires, the rod will buckle.

Dr. McGill reports scientists have tested the load-bearing capability of the human spine of cadavers. Testing the spine with the muscles removed (no guy wires), it can withstand a load of only twenty pounds. A properly supported spine of a young, healthy male; that is, with healthy bones and discs, muscles, tendons, and ligaments the spinal column can withstand a downward force of greater than two-thousand pounds without crushing or buckling!

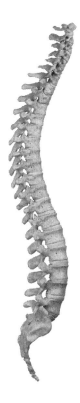

The spine

Chromosomes, genes, and DNA - Existing on the micro-level of our bodies are our chromosomes, with the twenty-thousand plus genes and the DNA contained in them. There are three billion base pairs in the language of DNA, which some have described as the body's *ultimate instruction guide.* If the string of DNA was published in book form it would consist of one-thousand books, each of one-thousand pages, and each page of a thousand letters. If you stretch out the DNA in a single cell, it would be 2.17 meters long. There are some 37.2 trillion cells in the average human body. If you were to stretch out *all* of the DNA in a human body, it is estimated to stretch across our solar system twice. Scientists have assigned varying huge estimates of distance, but you get the idea. More trivia: A single human hair is 40,000 times greater in diameter than a single strand of DNA.

Not too long ago, 98 percent of our DNA was referred to as non-coding junk (i.e., useless) DNA. Cell Biologist, Dr. Jay W. Shin, brings us up to date stating that the non-coding DNA produces RNA and is the control center of our DNA. The non-coding DNA incorporates thousands of important mechanisms such as combining proteins to achieve a functional end and operating as a GPS system to direct proteins where they need to go in a cell.

When a cell replicates, an incredible process is involved in which the three billion base pairs are copied, proofread, and errors corrected.

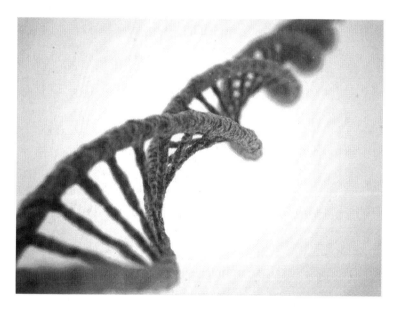

DNA model

The Brain - Dr. Paul David Nussbaum speaks of the human brain as "the single greatest, most magnificent system ever designed in the history of the universe, and it sits right between our ears!" He says it is capable of more than we can presently know and is deserving of a lifetime's dedication to health.

In his book, *What Is the Purpose of My Brain*? Dr. Nussbaum boldly explores its grand purpose:

> Perhaps God granted us a brain so that in his image, we could not only commune with him and his son Jesus Christ, but have the ability to believe, express our faith, and ultimately live our lives according to the teachings of Jesus Christ.

The human brain is a two to four-pound organ consisting of some 86 billion neurons (nerve cells) and comprised of sixty-percent fat. (We are all fatheads!) Recent scientific evidence suggests the brain produces thousands of new brain cells each day, and the rate of production can be increased by healthy eating and regular exercise, or the rate of production is slowed with an unhealthy lifestyle.

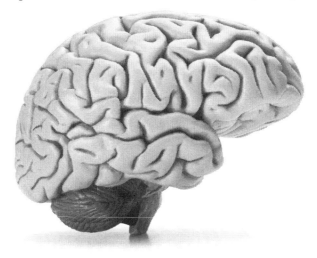

The brain

We are incredible beings! We have a lot to work with but unfortunately, sometimes things go wrong. There are genetic abnormalities, accidents, poor choices, and difficult circumstances that all impact our bodies and brains to reduce their strength, function, and performance. The good news is that we can often improve or reverse some negative outcomes. While we are "fearfully and wonderfully made," and the body has tremendous recovery potential, we need to act judiciously as wise managers of our lives.

The State of Our Nation's Health

A woman arrives at the emergency room experiencing a life-threatening diabetic crisis. During the early morning hours, a young man with a high alcohol blood level is transported in from a single car crash site. Later, a woman arrives by ambulance with signs and symptoms of a heart attack, and another gentleman is in cardiac arrest, with a paramedic administering CPR. All will be in good hands with the medical team, including David White, the attending emergency physician. (The same David we introduced earlier).

David has addressed many medical issues and injuries as a member of a medical team serving with Special Forces in Iraq; Navajo Nation, Chinle, Arizona; providing emergent care in two emergency departments in Central Pennsylvania; and a group practice for family and urgent care. David's observations led him to gain a new perspective. Too many of his patients' issues resulted from unhealthy lifestyle choices. A strong desire and plans for providing preventive medicine have since emerged, which is the antithesis of our current culture, one in which medical treatment typically trumps prevention.

We are an unhealthy nation, according to statistics gathered by the Centers for Disease Control and Prevention, American Cancer Society, American Diabetes Association, and American Heart Association.

Diabetes – It is no secret that diabetes is an epidemic in our nation, with more than 100 million people who are prediabetic or diabetic. Annually, more than a quarter million deaths are attributed to diabetes as the underlying or contributing cause. Children as young as four have been diagnosed with prediabetes or type 2 diabetes. Pain, suffering, and high financial costs are associated with the disease. The good news is that type 2 diabetes, which accounts for 90 to 95 percent of all diabetes, is a disease generated by lifestyle and is often reversible with a positive lifestyle change. Symptoms associated with type 1 diabetes can be mitigated with careful monitoring, regular exercise, and a healthy diet.

Obesity – A body mass index of 30 or higher is associated with a higher incidence of heart disease, stroke, type 2 diabetes, high blood pressure, a range of cancers, gallbladder disease, osteoarthritis, gout, sleep apnea, and asthma. Being overweight or obese correlates with inflammation in the body that contributes to the destruction of the cartilage in the knees and in the hips. To put things in perspective, a person who is 64 inches tall and weighs 175 is obese. A person who is 70 inches tall and weighs 210 is considered obese. (Exception: An athlete of the same height and weight may have a muscular physique with relatively low body fat. They would not be considered obese.) In 1960, thirteen percent of the population was obese. In 2017, almost thirty-eight percent of the adult population and twenty percent of adolescents were obese. In 2030, fifty percent of the population is expected to be obese.

Heart Disease – Every 40 seconds in the United States, a person has a heart attack—approximately 790,000 people yearly. The good news is that heart disease because it is a lifestyle-based disease, is largely preventable and may be reversible when it does occur. Dr. Caldwell Esselstyn is among many physicians who have had remarkable success in helping people reverse their coronary artery disease. His words, "Coronary artery disease is a toothless paper tiger that need never exist. If it does exist, it need not ever increase." His success in reversing coronary artery disease is tied to a radical change in diet—his patients were engaging in the whole food, plant-based side of the nutritional spectrum. Other physicians with similar success in preventing or reversing heart disease include Dr. Joel Fuhrman and Dr. Dean Ornish.

Lifestyle also impacts the health of the brain. Nationally recognized brain health expert clinical neuropsychologist Dr. Paul David Nussbaum is among the nation's forward-looking healthcare professionals who regularly write about the connection between our lifestyle choices, heart health, and the relationship between heart health and brain health. "What is good for the heart is good for the brain," says Dr. Nussbaum.

Alcohol and Drugs –Nearly 90,000 people die each year from alcohol-related causes, and we are currently struggling with an opioid epidemic in our nation. In 2022, there were 109,680 deaths associated with a drug overdose, with 79,770 deaths related to fentanyl and other synthetic opioids. Fentanyl is 50x more potent than heroin and 100x more potent than morphine.

Current research indicates that even the lower limit of alcohol consumption is associated with an increase in cancers. For example, low levels of alcohol consumption may raise the risk for breast and colorectal cancers, and a light level of consumption raises the risk for esophageal squamous cell carcinoma by 1.3x; for heavy drinking, it is an almost five-fold risk.

The picture becomes clear—much of our suffering through major disease is preventable or reversible. The key is a heart-level decision to live a healthy lifestyle through regular exercise, healthy eating, and restful sleep. It is critical to eliminate our exposure to toxins such as tobacco and the abuse of drugs and alcohol.

LIFESTYLE CHOICES OR GENES, AGE, AND GENDER?

Your age, your gender, and your family medical history can be discouraging if you hold to the belief that, when it comes to your health and longevity, your choices don't matter. If you're willing to join our emergency physician, Dr. David, in his desire to prevent disease, you recognize that you have much to say about your future health.

The book title by Dr. Walter M. Bortz, M.D., says it well: *We Live Too Short and Die Too Long.* A long, healthy, disability-free life is more an outcome of our lifestyle choices than our genes, gender, or age. Our bodies are made to live well beyond our current life expectancies, and the often physical and cognitive disabilities encountered in the latter decades of life are not a necessary part of aging.

SUPPORTING EVIDENCE

The Okinawa Study

The twenty-five-year Okinawa Study explains the unusual number of Okinawans living past one hundred years while continuing to be physically active and productive. Their healthy eating, being physically active, maintaining strong relationship ties, and having a strong spiritual foundation contribute to their vibrant longevity. The study concluded that if Americans lived like the Okinawans, we would have to close eighty percent of our coronary care units, one-third of our cancer wards, and a lot of our nursing homes.

Seventh-Day Adventists

A forty-year study of California Seventh-Day Adventists revealed a lifespan greater than that of non-Adventists and a lower risk of major diseases, including coronary heart disease and certain cancers. Their health and longevity were attributed to their lifestyle, strongly emphasizing their eating habits. Their diet was plant-based and included consuming nuts several times per week

Other Research Studies

Major diseases such as coronary artery disease, type 2 diabetes, and stroke are largely preventable. A cancer research study in 2008 conveys the same message as current research. Much of cancer is preventable:

Only 5–10% of all cancer cases can be attributed to genetic defects, whereas the remaining 90–95% have their roots in the environment and lifestyle. The lifestyle factors include cigarette smoking, diet (fried foods, red meat), alcohol, sun exposure, environmental pollutants, infections, stress, obesity, and physical inactivity. (*Pharmaceutical Research,* 2008 Sep; 25(9): 2097–2116)

The *Mayo Clinic, American Cancer Society,* Cancer *Prevention Research Center, MD Anderson Cancer Center, American Association for Cancer Research,* and *NIH National Cancer Institute* are among the many agencies across the United States that claim we can dramatically reduce the occurrence of cancers in our nation. It is not only that we can prevent significant disease, but we can often reverse the damage we have done to our bodies through poor lifestyle choices.

A Real Life Story

Meet Eula Weaver. At seventy-seven years old, she was frail and suffering from severe medical conditions, for which she was taking more than a dozen medications. She suffered a heart attack while undergoing a checkup at her doctor's office to add to her pain and woes. As she was about to be released from the hospital, her physician challenged her: "Eula, you have a choice. You can go home, go to bed, and have someone feed you with a spoon or start moving." Eula's response: "No one was going to feed me with a spoon! "

It was, however, much more difficult than she anticipated. Eula started a walking program, but it caused excruciating cramping in her legs after a few steps due to claudication—poor circulation in her lower legs. She was ready to give up until her son set up a meeting with the nutritionist, Nathan Pritikin. He advised her to keep walking despite the pain and radically change her poor eating habits.

Eula took his advice, ate healthily, and continued walking daily. It took eighteen months before she could jog a single lap, about 400 meters, around the local high school track. Her perseverance paid off. She entered the Senior Olympics at eighty-five, earning gold medals in the 800 and 1,500-meter runs. Five years later, a San Diego newspaper article heading read, "Eula Weaver Hangs Up

Competitive Racing Shoes at 90." She competed again and won two more medals.

When we live a healthy lifestyle, we generally feel better, look better, perform better, and are likelier to live a healthier, longer, disability-free life. In taking good care of our body and brain, we will

- be able to continue to do the things we love and enjoy.
- be at our best as we fulfill our life purpose.
- honor God by taking good care of His creation--OURSELVES.

Whether you are 25, 45, or 75, are you in the best condition to accomplish all you are about? Where do you want to go? What do you want to do when you get there? The effort you put into taking care of yourself will determine what you will be able to do, and, as we saw in Eula's life, it's never too late to make changes that will facilitate reaching our goals.

DID YOU KNOW?

Many of us hold to certain stereotypes about aging. Changes occur as we age, but a precipitous decline in body and brain health and conditioning is tied more to lifestyle factors than aging. Did you know that seventy percent of our reduction in strength over the decades is due not to aging but inactivity? A sensible exercise program would fortify and enrich the body and brain, slow the decline related to aging, and radically reduce the number of falls. Thirty percent of people over sixty-five and fifty percent of those over eighty fall in a single year.

- Most individuals are living far below their health, fitness, performance, quality of life and longevity potential.
- Health is much more a function of our day-to-day choices than of our genes, gender or age. A healthy lifestyle is associated with a healthier, longer life.
- God has built a tremendous recovery potential into our physical body—a capacity to reverse many of the effects of a disease, injury, misuse, and disuse.
- As we age, we will only be able to do what we "train" for.

THE INCREDIBLE RECOVERY POTENTIAL

OF THE AMAZING HUMAN BODY

You met Eula Weaver and now meet others who encountered and overcame significant barriers to health, performance, and longevity. The bad news is where we first find them; the good news is the rest of the story. The performance of these ordinary people doing extraordinary things demonstrates the tremendous recovery potential God has built into our amazing bodies.

Bad news for Barbara with very severe learning disabilities: As a child born with a most severe learning disability, Barbara Arrowsmith-Young could not understand logic or cause and effect. She could not tell time on a standard clock. If she placed her hand on a hot surface, she felt the pain but had no idea of its source. She was disconnected from the left side of her body and had a poor sense of the space and objects surrounding her, often bumping into things. She could not find her way around, even in places often visited, such as the home of her best friend. She said language was difficult and made no more sense to her than Lewis Carroll's *Jabberwocky* poem:

> Twas brillig, and the slithy toves
> Did gyre and gimble to the wabe;
> All mimsy were the borogoves,
> And the mome raths outgrabe.

<u>The rest of the story</u>: Barbara became determined to challenge her disabilities head-on. By creating novel ways of overcoming these barriers, she succeeded on all fronts. She can now think logically, comprehend and remember what she reads, has become in touch with the left side of her body, can tell time on a standard clock, and enjoys getting around with maps and her sense of direction rather than relying on a GPS. Barbara has completed a master's degree and opened a successful school in Canada for children with learning disabilities. Many of her ideas have been implemented in schools across Canada and the United States. She is the author of an inspiring book entitled *The Woman Who Changed Her Brain*.

Bad news for Ron when he had a stroke: Ron Dillon had a brain bleed while traveling on a plane. He was not expected to live but survived with a severe disability. He was told he would never walk, drive a car again, and be unable to work. A member of his stroke club had traveled around the country seeking treatment to regain the ability to walk. She warned Ron, "I have tried every resource and failed and cannot walk. It will be a cold day in Hell before you walk again!" Twelve years down the road, Ron was still not able to walk.

The rest of the story: Ron's rehabilitation center combined physical therapy with a robotic therapy system called the Quadriciser (www.quadriciser.com). It coordinates the movement of the arms and legs to simulate crawling and walking, resolving contractures along the way and affecting cross-patterning in the brain. It does the work of up to five persons, freeing the physical therapists to do what they do best. With this combination of interventions, Ron progressed to walking again. The first day he walked without a cane, he walked up to the woman from his stroke club and, reminding her of her gloomy forecast, said, "By the way, Hell just froze over." Ron was able to assume work duties as a volunteer and drive again.

Bad news for Johnny with type 2 diabetes: Johnny Rouse is a Hall of Fame college wrestling coach with two national team championships under his belt. Unfortunately, his type 2 diabetes destroyed his vision and required trans metatarsal amputations on both feet. At his peak weight, he was 340 pounds. At the time of his retirement from the public school system in 2001, Johnny selected a guaranteed ten-year income program "because I knew I wasn't going to live that long."

The rest of the story: After months on a whole-food, plant-based diet and regular exercise, he reported, "They said my vision would not improve, but I can see better. I can see a lot better!" In addition, he brought his average blood sugar to a non-diabetic level. As to his guaranteed ten-year retirement program, he said, "It's been seven years, and I'm feeling pretty good. So I think I chose the wrong program!" It is now closer to 18 years! He maintained a weight of around 182 pounds for many years, added and then lost a few pounds. His average blood sugar level remained in a normal range.

Bad news for Banana George, injured in a fall: After falling from a train at twenty, George Blair was told he may never walk again.

The rest of the story: Not only did George regain his ability to walk, but he took up water skiing in his 40s. Eventually, he mastered skiing barefoot and became a regular performer at Florida's Cyprus Gardens. "Banana George," as he became known, was featured in *The Guinness Book of Records*. His activities in his mid to late eighties included snowboarding, barefoot water skiing (holding the tow rope in his teeth), and working out at the local Gold's Gym. He was also a successful inventor and entrepreneur. You may have seen Banana George in TV ads or on Oprah or *Ripley's Believe It or Not*.

Bad news for William with heart issues: At age sixty-seven, Bill's father failed a routine exercise stress test. He experienced a potentially lethal heart arrhythmia one and a half minutes into the test. A heart medication was prescribed to control his abnormal heart rhythms.

The rest of the story: Over a period of weeks, he shook off his discouragement and began a walking routine. Walking led to jogging and eventually to compete in 10K races. In his eighties, William played ice hockey in a league in San Diego (he lied about his age to get on to the team), took up sky-diving, and bungee jumped out of a balloon. He worked full-time as an armed guard in a downtown bank, steadily improving his firearm testing scores over several years. In his mid-eighties, William became bored with jogging and 10K races. He began jogging up the steps at San Diego's Horton Plaza, up the stairs twenty times, 2,200 steps per workout!

Bad news for Sandy "destined" to an early death: Sandy had a family history of high cholesterol. In fact, all her extended family died young. She believed she was headed in the same direction. Even though she was not overweight, exercised regularly and worked with athletes professionally, her cholesterol was 248, her LDL was 173. Sandy was in her early thirties.

The rest of the story: Sandy began working with a health coach who recommended she drastically change her diet. Her physician was skeptical that it would make any difference, believing that the genetic factors were the sole cause of her high cholesterol. The physician was wrong. Her nutritional choices lowered her cholesterol to 180, with an LDL of 120. She noted that she was no longer tired in the afternoon and had increased energy. Most importantly, she was not headed for an early death. She felt a tremendous cloud was lifted and was tearful as she thought about enjoying her family for many years into the future.

The takeaway from the lives of these heroes: As athletes train for their respective sports, you and I would do well to be training for life, regardless of our age or the condition in which we find ourselves today.

Three lifestyle factors—exercise, nutrition, and sleep—are

among those that contribute toward fortifying the body and brain. To review: Being fortified means that the body and brain's physical structure, anatomy, and physiology are healthy and sound. When your brain accelerates the production of new brain cells due to exercise and good nutrition, the brain is fortified with the new brain cells, which go to work to improve cognitive performance. To be fortified is also to enrich the body and brain to perform at their highest level physically and cognitively. For example, if you learn a new physical skill, you also develop new connections (synapses) in the brain. If you are training for muscular strength and power, you are better able to carry out the physical and mental tasks of your day.

A RATIONALE FOR EXERCISE

Amy was in a discussion with two of our grandchildren, Sydney and Brannen, ages four and six. A question about death and heaven surfaced. Sydney said she didn't want to die and go to heaven. When Grammy asked why she didn't want to go to heaven, Syd said, "Because my eyes would be closed, and that would be boring." Brannen responded by saying that if you don't want to die, you have to exercise. He added, referring to Bill, "PopPop exercises *a lot,* and it is a good thing because he is *very old*!"

Exercise does not guarantee a long life, but exercise is dose-related to longevity, health, and a level of independence and function in the latter years. In 2007, the American College of Sports Medicine and the American Medical Association, with the support of the Office of the Surgeon General, considered these benefits when it launched a program entitled "Exercise is Medicine" (exerciseismedicine.org).

Our bodies are made for movement. Research from the Harvard School of Public Health underscores the positive impact regular exercise has on health and longevity. Exercisers, in general, appreciate a better quality of life and a longer life than their peer couch potatoes. The Cooper Institute, based upon almost forty-eight years of research, has found people could extend their life expectancy by six to nine years by engaging in regular exercise. The benefits of exercise have been recognized for a long time

From HIPPOCRATES (460 – 357 BC), the ancient Greek physician, labeled "the father of medicine":

> If we could give every individual the right amount of nourishment and exercise, not too little and not too much, we would have found the safest way to health.

Sudden death is more common in those who are naturally

fat than in the lean. From MARTIN LUTHER (1483 – 1546)

> I do not deny that medicine is a gift of God, nor do I refuse to acknowledge science in the skill of many physicians; but, take the best of them, how far are they from perfection? A sound regimen produces excellent effects. When I feel indisposed, by observing a strict diet and going to bed early, I generally manage to get round again, that is if I can keep my mind tolerably at rest. I have no objection to the doctors acting upon certain theories, but, at the same time, they must not expect us to be the slaves of their fancies.
>
> I expect that exercise and change of air do more good than all their purgings and bleedings; but when we do employ medical remedies, we should be careful to do so under the advice of a judicious physician.

Studies have suggested that regular, moderate exercise can dramatically reduce the risk for heart disease, stroke, breast and other forms of cancer, diabetes, dementia (Alzheimer's and vascular), and fractures from falls. Only three and one-half percent of the adult population meets the minimum exercise requirements set forth by the American College of Sports Medicine, American Heart Association, and American Cancer Society. The minimum standard is thirty minutes of moderate aerobic exercise five times per week (or three twenty-minute sessions of higher intensity), two whole-body strength training sessions per week (about twenty minutes each), and regular stretching. Recently, there has been an emphasis on adding skilled activities requiring balance, coordination, and agility, such as racquet sports.

Exercise directly impacts the brain. For example, intense exercise elevates a brain chemical (the fancy name is *brain-derived neurotrophic factor*) that stimulates the production of new brain cells in the hippocampus area of the brain. The hippocampus is involved in learning, memory, and spatial navigation. Studies with older adults have demonstrated that a progressive exercise program increases brain volume in the hippocampus with an associated improvement in cognition.

Regular exercise offers a brain benefit to persons with Parkinson's by increasing dopamine production, a chemical critical to physical and mental function. Exercise also stimulates the production of a chemical that reduces the occurrence of panic attacks in those prone to have them. (An excellent reference to these and other encouraging facts is the book *Spark: The Revolutionary New Science of Exercise and the Brain* by John J. Ratey, M.D.)

A RATIONALE FOR ENJOYING THE POWER OF GOOD NUTRITION

Exercise promotes health, but what about nutrition? We have already presented evidence from the twenty-five-year Okinawa Study and the 40 years invested in the Adventist Studies. We could also begin to build a case from the Old and New Testaments regarding the wisdom of following a plant-based diet.

> Then God said, "I give you every seed-bearing plant on the face of the whole earth and every tree that has fruit with seed in it. They will be yours for food. And to all the beasts of the earth and all the birds of the air and all the creatures that move on the ground—everything that has the breath of life in it—I give every green plant for food." And it was so. (Gen. 1:29-30)

In the 6th century BC, Daniel, on behalf of himself and his friends, petitioned the king's steward to be allowed to put aside the king's delicacies and instead to consume vegetables and water.

> "Test your servants for ten days; let us be given vegetables to eat and water to drink. Then let our appearance and the appearance of the youths who eat the king's food be observed by you, and deal with your servants according to what you see." So he listened to them in this matter, and tested them for ten days. At the end of ten days it was seen that they were better in appearance and fatter in flesh than all the youths who ate the king's food. (Daniel 1:12-15)

From a biblical perspective, however, it is not that certain foods are forbidden. In the New Covenant, dietary restrictions regarding eating specific animals were lifted. However, the point of the text quoted here is not a diet but the inclusion of all cultures, nations, and races in the plan of salvation. Peter had a vision of "all kinds of four-footed animals . . . and birds of the air," He heard a voice, "Rise, Peter; kill and eat." Peter protested, saying he had never eaten anything "common or unclean." He was told, "What God has cleansed you must not call common." Further, the Scriptures teach: "The man who eats everything must not look down on him who does not, and the man who does not eat everything must not condemn the man who does, for God has accepted him." (Romans 14:3)

The question is not whether a type of food is permitted but whether it is wise to consume certain foods, especially with the frequency and large meal portions common to Western nations. Do the words of Paul, speaking with God's authority, apply here? "Everything is permissible for me—but not everything is beneficial. Everything is permissible for me—but I will not be mastered by anything." (1 Corinthians 6:12)

There is an avalanche of nutritional information—both good and bad—available in the printed and electronic media. There are conflicting views and ongoing debates about what constitutes a healthy diet. Up-to-date, sound research cuts through the confusion and refutes false claims. We will revisit this in the next chapter.

A RATIONALE FOR SLEEP, WONDERFUL SLEEP

We Americans tend to be sleep-deprived people. A lack of restful sleep takes a toll on our bodies and brains.

- Extended periods of sleep deficit destroy brain cells.

- A sleep-deprived person's driving is as impaired as that of a person driving under the influence of alcohol.

- Getting quality sleep is key to maintaining good health. It's impossible to effectively manage stress when you're tired. Proper sleep is critical to brain function.

- Long-term sleep deficits affect your reaction time, judgment—even your short-term memory and vision.

- Tired people are more moody and aggressive.

- A person getting regular, restful sleep will generally

awaken refreshed and rested each morning after passing through the normal cycles of sleep during the night.

- Most adults require at least 8 hours of sleep each night; some of us require a little more. More than 9 hours of sleep is associated with poorer health. People who sleep less than 6 hours or more than 9 hours a night have a higher incidence of type 2 diabetes.

- The notorious alarm clock awakens most of us before we have gotten the sleep we need. Most people stay up too late, missing those hours before midnight which has the most restorative potential.

Good things happen in our bodies while we sleep

- Waste products deposited in the brain during waking hours are flushed out especially during sleep—not through the brain's blood vessels, but the cerebral-spinal fluid being pumped around the blood vessels through the brain.

- Injured tissue heals more rapidly.

- Muscle tissue is "injured" during strength training, then repaired while muscle size increases.

- Cell division is faster while we sleep. The cells of the skin, intestinal lining and blood are constantly being replaced.

- Erythrocytes are the red blood cells, and we have about 25 trillion of them. Red blood cells have a lifespan of only 3 to 4 months, replaced at a rate of three million per second!

- Liver processes speed up.

- Your central nervous system is rejuvenated.

- The output of growth hormone is increased.

- Your brain is at work transferring what is stored as short-term memory to long-term memory.

As you have seen, the evidence suggests there is good news—our choices matter. However, we may encounter obstacles to pursuing a healthy lifestyle. There is a strong rationale for taking good care of the body. Such self-management increases the likelihood of living a long, disability-free, active life. Much can be said about what constitutes the lifestyle that carries the body and brain to its full potential. As we continue our discussion, we will offer evidence-based guidelines, emphasizing some detailed instructions for exercise, nutrition, and sleep.

CHAPTER 7

HEALTH THROUGH EXERCISE, NUTRITION, AND SLEEP

EXERCISE

Dr. Kenneth Cooper, founder of the Cooper Aerobics Center and the father of aerobics, was once asked what is the best form of exercise. His response: "The kind you are willing to do." Dr. Cooper firmly believed that running three miles a day enabled him to keep up with his busy schedule. Dr. Cooper is still busy and, no surprise, still exercising—even in his late eighties.

Even if we're not at the same level as Dr. Cooper, exercise is still critical to maintaining a strong, healthy body. For all of us, the ideal exercise program is multi-dimensional and brings a return on investment by contributing to each major area of life— better health, the energy to get everything done that matters to us, more restful and adequate sleep, and facilitating optimal performance both in our work and recreational pursuits.

THINK ABOUT IT: If you don't believe you have enough time for exercise in your already jam-packed schedule, consider the benefits listed above. Making exercise a top priority may increase your ability to accomplish your goals.

THE BENEFITS OF EXERCISE

Our bodies are made for movement. Immediate goals of regular exercise include the following:

- Achieve and maintain full, unrestricted movement without pain.

- Build overall endurance and stamina.

- Develop skilled movement with balance, agility, and coordination for work, recreational and primary day-to-day tasks that involve squatting and lifting, trunk and whole-body rotation, single leg movement (which includes walking), and multi-directional pulling and pushing movements.

- Train for increased explosive strength referred to as power (strength with acceleration) in the upper body, lower body, and core. (Muscular power may be the best predictor of quality of life for the latter years; even more predictive than aerobic fitness or muscular strength.)

- Maintain a sharp brain, with the ability for short-term memory, long-term memory, ability to learn, capacity to remember and recall what is learned, problem-solving ability and ability to focus and concentrate. Regular body exercise, especially bouts of intense exercise, plus novel and complex cognitive learning, in addition to truly healthy eating all contribute to brain health and the postponement or reduction of the risk for dementia, including Alzheimer's.

Wondering where to begin? Remember, "the best kind of exercise is the kind you are willing to do." For starters, if you are healthy, start moving! As a start, begin walking, increasing your time, tempo, and frequency week-by-week. Build up to the recommended eight to ten thousand steps per day. Commit to regular activity across a range of types of exercise. Incorporating all exercise areas into a lifestyle may seem daunting, but many activities simultaneously address multiple areas.

A LOOK AT FIVE TYPES OF EXERCISE

- Flexibility
- Strength
- Skilled movement
- Aerobic (cardio-respiratory)
- Brain-specific exercise (a wide range of novel, challenging learning activities across multiple areas of intelligence)

Flexibility

Daily stretching brings several lasting benefits. It enables your body to work better. Short stretches take the tissue to the elastic phase, from which the muscle returns to its pre-stretch length. Longer stretches, stretching for twenty to thirty seconds or longer, take the tissue to the plastic phase, enabling the muscle to remodel to a new length. Except for stretching the lower back tissues (see additional notes below) and possibly the hamstring muscles, stretching the muscles helps with mobility, balance, and overall physical performance and helps reduce the risk of injury. Tight hamstrings can work to the benefit of some, but not all, athletes.

Taking the time to stretch each day brings several changes. The muscle adds new micro-units and connective tissue at the muscle ends, increasing its overall length. The connective tissue surrounding the muscle fibers and entire muscles becomes longer, better organized, and less stiff. Elastic proteins in the muscles and tendons increase, making them less prone to tearing. There is an increase in the production of molecules that provide lubrication for the joints and connective tissue.

Additional Notes on Stretching

According to Dr. Stuart McGill, the lower back is more about stability than flexibility and muscle endurance than sheer muscle strength, so exercise accordingly; stretch the lower back to the extent of the range of motion required in your daily and sports activities. As a side comment, a great way to injure your back is to sit all day without taking frequent mobility and stretch breaks. Another back destroyer is doing sit-ups. Still, another is bending and twisting as you lift an object from the floor or simply lifting an object immediately after sitting for an extended period.

Stretches of long duration done immediately before a sports competition—more than twenty-thirty seconds per stretch—are thought by some experts to hinder performance by reducing elastic recoil and increasing the risk of injury from joint laxity. It is also possible to go to the extreme of overstretching muscles, resulting in pain and loss of strength and performance.

Stretching worked muscles between sets of a strength training exercise quickly restores the muscle to its normal length and shortens recovery time for the next set.

Types of Stretches

Static stretches - take a muscle to the place of tension and hold the stretch position for a designated number of seconds (typically at least thirty seconds—for example, facing and leaning against a wall with one foot back and heel down to stretch the calf).

Active stretches - move a joint through its range of motion and hold briefly (several repetitions, typically for two to three seconds each).

Dynamic stretches - actively lengthen a muscle by applying force and body momentum (for example, stepping into a forward lunge, or performing a squat with the hands behind the head).

PNF stretches - work a muscle against light resistance for a few seconds, followed by a stretch of the same muscle.

Not including regular stretching in your exercise program may result in a loss of range of motion; increased risk for injury and related-pain; excess wear in the joints; limitations in activity.

We Are Body/Brain Sculptors

God is the Creator, and we are the body and brain sculptors. Bill: I remember as a kid squishing up my face in response to express disapproval, and my mother saying, "If you keep making that face, it is going to stay that way." If that is true about a face, it is more of the body. We are a big lump of clay because the body tends to take on the shape and posture that we assume daily. For example, if you sit over a computer with your head forward, shoulders rounded, and pelvis rotated forward, it will create muscle imbalances that lead to injury and pain.

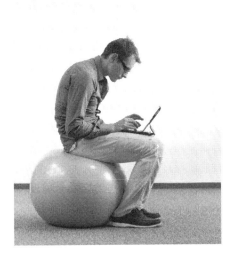

Do you sit for long periods each day? What is your posture? Even the best posture, sitting with a neutral spine, shoulders square, and head aligned, is unsuitable for the body if you sit for extended periods. Worse, of course, is the posture depicted above in the photo of the man on the stability ball. Back experts, such as Dr. Stuart M. McGill, suggest that after fifty minutes or so of sitting, we should frequently stand and move about.

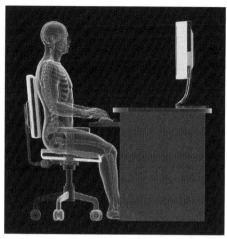

A bent-over walking posture in old age is often a function of inactivity, and negative habits of movement, lying, standing, and sitting. For most of us, it need not be a condition of aging.

Do you have posture imbalances? By correctly rolling (referred to as self-myofascial release; see photo illustration below), then stretching tight, overactive muscles (such as the hip flexors), and activating and strengthening the inhibited, lengthened opposing muscles (such as the gluteus maximus), balance can be restored. Physical therapists, chiropractors, and exercise physiologists with corrective exercise training are resource people who can address muscle imbalances.

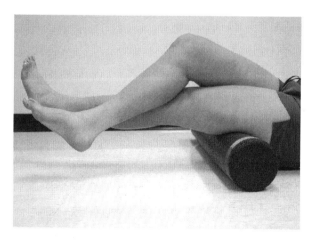

In addition to the rounded shoulder example, other muscle imbalances are indicated if the shoulder blades are winged out; feet are turned outward; knees are turned inward with our feet flattened;

we lean when walking or standing; hips are tilted backward on our femurs (large bones of the thigh) flattening out the curve in the lower back, or tilted forward on the femurs causing an excess curve of the lower back; head, hips or shoulders are rotated clockwise or counter-clockwise; one hip or shoulder is higher than its opposite; or the head is tilted to one side.

If during the day the hip flexors (see the illustration below) are tight and overactive from sitting, the opposite muscle, the gluteus maximus (your sit-upon muscle) will likely be inhibited, lengthened and weak. Many muscles address the stability and movements related to the hips and to the stability of the spine. Because the body is a single orchestra of closely-related instruments, an imbalance or abnormality or injury in an element will affect what is below and above. A problem in a hip muscle may result in plantar fasciitis, causing pain on the bottom of the foot—typically near the heel, or knee, or back or shoulder pain. In choosing a coach, trainer, chiropractor or physical therapist, choose wisely. Not all are created equal. A personal trainer whose preparation is limited to a weekend personal training course is not a good choice.

Hip Flexors that are tight (for example, from sitting for long periods during the day) means that the glutes will likely be inhibited, weak, and lengthened.

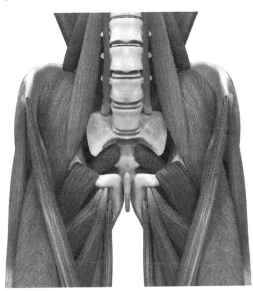

The hip flexors are the ones on either side of the spine thatconnect o the femur in the thigh, and the muscles next to them connecting the inner surface and crest of the hip bones to the femur. (The femur is not visible.)

The gluteus maximus, illustrated below, is the largest muscle in the body. It is also one that visibly atrophies and weakens with age when one is sedentary.

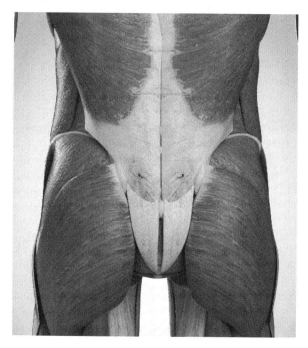

If you have none of the concerns described, move forward with a sensible, progressive and comprehensive exercise program covering at least the five areas to follow.

Strength – (Resistance) Training

Training to increase muscle, tendon, ligament, and bone strength is critical if you want to be highly functioning, doing the things you love and are called to do throughout life. The larger percentage of those who become physically dependent in their 8th and 9th decades are so not because of their chronic medical conditions but due to muscle and bone weakness (sarcopenia and osteopenia/osteoporosis). Keep in mind to progress slowly in strengthening muscles through resistance training. Muscles strengthen faster than the tendons that connect muscles to bones. Progressing too rapidly may result in a tendon injury.

If you are not familiar with the exercises listed over the next several pages, go to *YouTube* for video illustrations. Exercising to build or strengthen your muscles involves creating resistance via weights dumbbells, barbells, kettlebells, sandbells, ViPR, straps (TRX, or straps with rings), machines (plates, weight stack or compressed air), rubber bands, or working your body against gravity.

Doing pushups, in which you are lifting your body weight off the floor, is an example of using your own body weight. Other examples of body weight exercise include lunges, wall-ball squats, prisoner squats, jumping, pull-ups, power walking, jogging or running.

Strength training makes it easier to do everyday chores such as carrying laundry or groceries and improves life's primary functional movements—squatting and lifting, pushing, pulling, rotation, and movement on one foot (which includes walking).

The traditional strength machines you find in most gyms determine your path and range of motion and do not necessarily require the use of stabilizing muscles in the ankles, knees, core, and shoulders. They may increase strength while compromising performance and stability. They can have their place but should not be relied on primarily. Studies have shown a decline in balance for men with the exclusive use of traditional strength machines for exercise. Machines that use cables with handles—for example, many of the types of cable equipment manufactured by Free Motion and Keiser—are superior to the traditional strength machines because they require the use of the stabilizing muscles. Each type of equipment has its advantages and disadvantages. These issues are addressed in-depth in research projects available on the web.

With multi-directional resistance movements with the ViPR, cables, rubber bands, kettlebells and dumbbells you determine the path and range of motion and typically engage the stabilizing muscles. For example, if you stand and execute a pulling or pushing motion against the resistance of bands, you must use the core (including hip, abdominal and back muscles), ankles and knees to maintain your stance.

Current research suggests the best predictor of how you will function physically in the decades to come is your level of muscular power. Power is strength times acceleration, explosive strength.

A man tripped and fell on a sidewalk. Tripping on a raised section of concrete, he instinctively stepped forward to catch himself. He had the coordination and quickness to prevent a fall but lacked the explosive power in his leg and hip to stop his forward momentum. His leg gave way, and his face met the pavement. Preventing a fall in this instance is not unlike the power demonstrated by the gymnast who sticks her landing in the dismount from the balance beam.

Power training combines speed with maximum strength. It is

designed for developing the kind of explosive strength required for a variety of life activities, plus a host of athletic activities such as sprinting, jumping, kicking, punching, and throwing. Power training exercises include medicine ball throws, jump squats, and power cleans. Plyometric training involves a particular form of power exercise in which the muscle is loaded in a lengthening contraction (as dropping down to a quarter or half-squat), followed immediately by a shortening contraction (as leaping into the air from the quarter or half-squat position).

Gymnasts who "stick" a landing in various events have trained for this kind of power. Power training, especially plyometrics, should not be attempted until you have conditioned for an extended period of muscle, endurance, and strength training. Exercise that strengthens your muscles also strengthens your bones because bones restructure along lines of force.

Resistance exercise should begin with an eight to ten-week adaptation phase (relatively low intensity and resistance) to prevent injury and facilitate progress. As mentioned, muscles develop faster than tendons, so the adaptation phase helps to prevent unnecessary injury to the tendons. Training should be progressive, allowing you to gradually increase strength until you reach your maximum potential or goal strength.

As an athlete's training program should be tailored to the demands of the sport, so training for the non-athlete should be tailored to the demands of day-to-day life. Strength should be developed along the lines of the functional movements combining our everyday activities, including pushing and pulling, rotational movement, movement on one foot (in walking, we spend 68% of our time on one foot), and squatting and lifting. As we age, we will only be able to do what we train for!

Strength Training for the Core

Current research suggests the best predictor of how you will function physically in the decades to come is your level of muscular power. Power is strength times acceleration, explosive strength.

A man tripped and fell on a sidewalk. Tripping on a raised section of concrete, he instinctively stepped forward to catch himself. He had the coordination and quickness to prevent a fall but lacked the explosive power in his leg and hip to stop his forward momentum.

His leg gave way, and his face met the pavement. Preventing a fall in this instance is not unlike the power demonstrated by the gymnast who sticks her landing in the dismount from the balance beam.

Power training combines speed with maximum strength. It is designed for developing the kind of explosive strength required for a variety of life activities, plus a host of athletic activities such as sprinting, jumping, kicking, punching, and throwing. Power training exercises include medicine ball throws, jump squats, and power cleans. Plyometric training involves a particular form of power exercise in which the muscle is loaded in a lengthening contraction (as dropping down to a quarter or half-squat), followed immediately by a shortening contraction (as leaping into the air from the quarter or half-squat position).

Gymnasts who "stick" a landing in various events have trained for this kind of power. Power training, especially plyometrics, should not be attempted until you have conditioned for an extended period of muscle, endurance, and strength training. Exercise that strengthens your muscles also strengthens your bones because bones restructure along lines of force.

Resistance exercise should begin with an eight to ten-week adaptation phase (relatively low intensity and resistance) to prevent injury and facilitate progress. As mentioned, muscles develop faster than tendons, so the adaptation phase helps to prevent unnecessary injury to the tendons. Training should be progressive, allowing you to gradually increase strength until you reach your maximum potential or goal strength.

As an athlete's training program should be tailored to the demands of the sport, so training for the non-athlete should be tailored to the demands of day-to-day life. Strength should be developed along the lines of the functional movements combining our everyday activities, including pushing and pulling, rotational movement, movement on one foot (in walking, we spend 68% of our time on one foot), and squatting and lifting. As we age, we will only be able to do what we train for.

McGill Crunch: With one knee bent and one straight, with hands in the lower back to maintain the lumbar curve (or place a small rolled towel), and with your head in line with your torso, lift your shoulder blades slightly off the floor. (After completing half of your repetitions, reverse the position of the legs). Dr. Stuart McGill does *not* recommend the typical way of doing a crunch of placing your hands behind the head while bending the head forward.

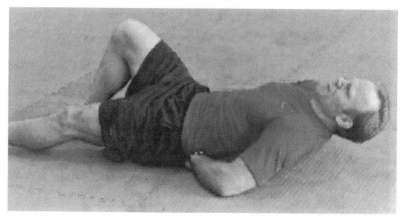

Bird Dog: Hands directly below your shoulders, and your knees directly below the hips, extend opposite arm and leg. Return to the start position and repeat with the same leg and arm. Switch to other leg and arm and repeat. (Keep your hips level, and when you lift the leg do not lift it above the height of the hips).

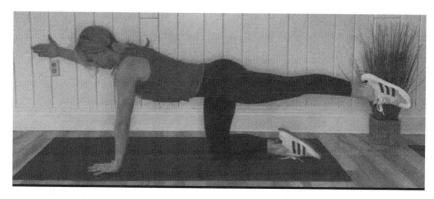

Stabilization exercises allow you to maintain joint and/or postural positions over a designated number of seconds. Strength training allows you to improve your ability to exert muscular force as in lifting a weight. Power training increases explosive strength: as in jumping or throwing activity. Examples of thousands of exercises of each category can be found on the web—e.g., on YouTube.com. The side plank, illustrated on the next page, is an excellent core strength stabilization exercise. Note that the elbow is *directly* below the shoulder, and the body is in perfect straight alignment.

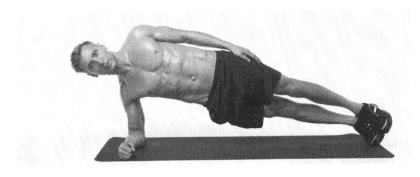

Not including strength training in your exercise program may result in a loss of muscle mass and strength (25% loss by age 65), and loss of bone mass (increased fracture risk); loss of muscle mass and strength with slower metabolism and fat weight gain. Balance is negatively affected by increased muscle atrophy.

Skilled Movement

Skilled movement includes training for improved balance, agility, coordination, and quickness of reflexes, and is very beneficial for both body *and* brain.

- *Balance* is your ability to maintain your center of mass over your stance of support, either while standing or in motion.

- *Agility* is the ability to quickly change speed and direction, moving forward or backward, side-to-side, or diagonally with proper posture.

- *Coordination* involves activity in which the different parts of the body move in harmony with smoothness and efficiency.

- *Quickness* is defined as the ability to react with an immediate change of position and movement with appropriate strength in an activity.

All four skills are basic for activities such as racquet sports, dance, skiing, snowboarding, floor exercise and the vault in gymnastics, team sports such as softball, basketball and soccer, and the martial arts. Agility, balance, coordination, and quickness enable you to avoid collisions with people or shopping carts, bicycles, or other objects unexpectedly and suddenly coming your way.

Pictured on the next page is actor, model, and fitness professional, Stephanie Haff. The illustrated pose combines balance, mobility, and flexibility.

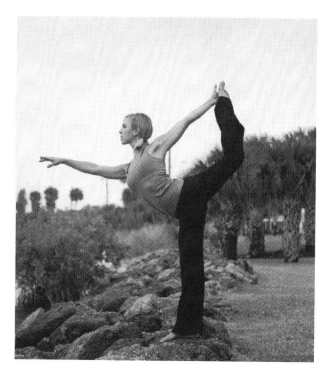

Regarding balance, suppose you are walking down the sidewalk, and someone gently bumps you from behind. You rock forward a little, adjusting at your ankles to realign your body over your base of support. If you were bumped a bit harder, you would rock forward and back from the hips, realigning your body over its base of support. Bumped harder still, you would step forward to keep from falling. If, in stepping forward, you lacked power in your leg and hip, you could fall on your face. Balance is a complex skill, with training requiring feedback from your muscles, joints, vision, and inner ear. Balance training improves with training for coordination, agility, muscular strength, and power.

As we age, we tend to shrink the circle of daily activity, resulting in an unnecessary physical decline. Seventy percent of our reduction in strength over the decades is not due to aging but inactivity. Over thirty percent of people over sixty-five and over fifty percent of those over eighty fall in a year. Research indicates the risk of a fall increases significantly if you cannot stand on one foot for more than thirty seconds; the risk increases for an injurious fall if you cannot stand on one foot for only five seconds (a fall that likely sends you to the emergency room).

Recently, twenty-seven men and women living independently with an average age of eighty-three were assessed for their level of function at the start of an eight-week exercise program. One of the assessments was a simple, stand-on-one-foot balance test. No participant could balance on one foot for more than two seconds. Despite their independent status, each was at risk for injurious falls.

As we age, we can only do what we train for. Tai Chi, a Chinese martial art, has been shown to improve balance by fifty percent in three months with just two training sessions per week. Certain forms of dance and the martial arts practice will improve balance and coordination.

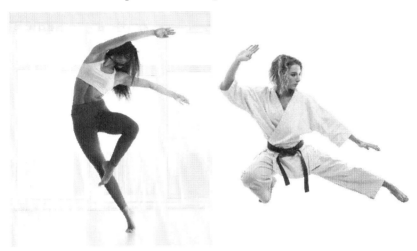

Not including skilled activity in your exercise program may result in a loss of balance, coordination, and agility as you age. As stated, as you age you will only be able to do what you train for. Skilled movement activity allows you to maintain flexibility, range of motion, and mobility.

Aerobic (Cardiorespiratory) Exercise

Aerobic activities are those sustaining an increased heart rate and breathing rate during the activity. They improve heart and brain function, increase your stamina, help you manage your weight, and reduce your risk for a major disease. Interval training (light to moderate, alternated with intense) is best for weight loss.

A minimum recommendation for aerobic exercise is thirty minutes per day, five days per week. Aim to build up to 45 minutes per day, at least 5 days per week. An example of interval training is to do a two-minute warm-up at a light intensity, then alternate between high intensity and low intensity or resting, and finish with a light cool-down.

Recently, persons diagnosed with congestive heart failure were put on an interval training program alternating the intensity phase with complete rest. The result was improved heart function and fewer episodes of arrhythmias.

If you are over fifty-five years of age, have been sedentary for a long time, or have a heart problem, get your physician's OK before venturing into such a program. If you have had a cardiac event or are diagnosed with a heart problem, enroll in a cardiac rehabilitation program. (With a referral by a cardiologist, your thirty-six sessions may be covered by your insurance.)

If your goal is to lose weight and you choose to engage in steady-state (steady pace throughout) rather than interval training, exercise in the "fat-burning zone." Your breathing will increase, often pausing to take breaths between words. If you are so out of breath that you can't carry on a conversation, you are burning mostly sugar instead of fat.

Aerobic exercise causes some important changes to take place in the skeletal muscles: [1]The energy-producing factories, the mitochondria, increase in number by as much as fifty percent in three months. [2]The myoglobin, which carries and delivers oxygen in the muscle, increases. [3]The capillary beds become richer with more tiny blood vessels are extended from your existing capillaries. [4]There is an increase in aerobic enzymes, further facilitating the efficient production of energy. All of this translates into greater energy and endurance for doing all the things you need and love to do.

Not including aerobic activity in my exercise program may result in a loss of ten-percent of aerobic capacity for each decade after age thirty; loss of stamina; elevated risk for cancer, heart disease, diabetes, and stroke; loss of brain volume and cognitive performance; greater risk for dementia.

Incorporating all areas of exercise into a lifestyle may seem daunting, but many activities address multiple areas simultaneously. Examples are the martial arts, dance, and racquet sports.

Brain building through Brain-Specifc Exercise

In his book entitled, *Save Your Brain,* Dr. Paul David Nussbaum discusses the five things you must do to keep your mind young and sharp. He presents a clear, convincing case for preventing memory loss, improving brain performance, and increasing mental fitness by implementing a brain-healthy lifestyle that includes good nutrition, physical activity, spirituality, socialization, and mental stimulation.

The emphasis on mental stimulation is the pursuit of novel, challenging, and complex learning activities. It engages both basic brain function and higher brain function. The components of both levels—basic and higher cognitive function—all work together and therefore need to be trained in concert through regular practice of various combinations of expression. That is, you do not train an area of brain function in isolation from other areas of function.

Suppose you set a goal to improve your balance in the bodily-kinesthetic area of intelligence. Balance is not addressed in isolation as though is stand on its own. Incorporate a complex activity into your plans such as dance or the martial arts. In these, balance is developed in the context of skilled movements that include not only balance per se, but also coordination, agility, quickness, flexibility, strength, power, proprioception, memory, and concentration. With dance, of course, you benefit from the addition of music and rhythm. You could build a case for also tapping into spatial, intrapersonal, and interpersonal intelligences in your training plans.

Basic cognitive function includes memory, concentration, and sensory processing via hearing, seeing, smelling, touching, tasting

Higher cognitive function (including the multiple-intelligence categories of Dr. Howard Gardner referred to earlier) includes executive function, problem-solving, academic learning; language; interpersonal intelligence; intrapersonal inteligence(the capacity to make sound decisions fed by an understanding of self, and the awareness, and implications, of moment-by-moment emotions and feeling responses); artistic-spatial; navigation-spatial; bodily-kinesthetic (skilled movement); and musical. There are other areas of intelligence Dr. Gardner has researched that we will not take time address here. We add chronemic, *timing,* as an area of intelligence which we believe deserves special notice for its place in interpersonal communication, entertainment, skilled work activities, sports, and daily life in general. The area of the brain referred to as the *thalamus* has a role in *timing* as it links with attention, alertness, awareness, perception, and movement.

Examples of activities to engage the brain include mind-challenging games such as Soduku, bridge, chess, Scrabble, Upwords, Quirkle, and many others; puzzles of all kinds; critical problem-solving; new, challenging learning or activity in any single area or combined areas of intelligence; academic studies and serious reading; web-based brain exercises; memorization; music composition; writing a story or poem; finding your way around by following a map; and activities requiring the development of physical skills (fine motor or large muscle skills). The idea is to engage in a wide range of brain activity and not limit yourself to a single category.

Not engaging in challenging, novel, complex brain activity plus regular physical exercise may result in a reduced cognitive function and greater risk for dementia.

A NUTRITION PRIMER

Exercise promotes health, but what about nutrition? In the previous chapter, we began to build a case from the Old and New Testaments regarding the wisdom of following a plant-based diet.

An avalanche of confusing nutrition information is available in the printed and electronic media. There are conflicting views and ongoing debates about what constitutes a healthy diet. Up-to-date, sound research cuts through the confusion and refutes many false claims.

What you can take to the Bank from the Nutritional Research

Ill-advised foods include those laden with salt or sugar; "white foods" such as white rice and white flour in bread, cereals, pancakes, and waffles; processed foods, including those with a long list of hard-to-pronounce ingredients; red meat, processed meat (and some say meat in general, including chicken).

Often, the advice to limit, rather than eliminate, these foods is either the food industry weighing in on their behalf or is a compromise based on the assumption people are not willing to forsake them entirely. How much poison are you willing to eliminate from your diet?

Two studies on meat, heart disease, and cancer are from 37,698 men from the Health Professionals Follow-up Study (HPFS) and 83,644 women from the Nurses' Health Study (NHS). After adjustment for multiple risk factors, daily eating an additional serving of meat was associated with a sixteen percent increase in the risk of cardiovascular mortality and a ten-percent increased risk of death from cancer.

Recommended

Whole, nutrient-dense food: unprocessed fruits and vegetables plus nuts, seeds, whole grains, beans, and legumes are associated with a reduced risk for significant disease and disability-free longevity. Studies on heart prevention and reversal conducted by Doctors Caldwell Esselstyn, Hans Diehl, Joel Fuhrman, and Dean Ornish support the consumption of whole, nutrient-dense food. Additional research supporting the health benefits of whole, nutrient-dense foods (as they say, "foods that have no face or a mother") are found in The China Study, the Adventist Health Study 2, and the Okinawa

Centenarian Study. One of the factors associated with centenarians in the Okinawa Study was a practice called "hara hucchi bu," which involves eating till you are only eighty percent full—consuming about forty percent less than consumed by North Americans. Okinawa boasts the greatest number in the world of centenarians per capita. The study found that, in general, the Okinawa centenarians are not just old. They are high-functioning people not burdened with the disability you might expect of the old, old, old.

Recent research indicates certain foods prevent the growth of early, small cancer tumors by inhibiting angiogenesis (the formation of new blood vessels in the tumor). These foods include, but are not limited to, soy extract, parsley, berries, soy, garlic, red grapes, citrus, lavender, green tea, turmeric, and tea. The effectiveness of these foods is possibly related to the fact that the blood vessels in tumors are inferior and, therefore, more vulnerable to destruction or are less likely to form.

Another series of studies addresses gene expression. Genes can be good or bad in their impact on the body, but this is not the end of the story. Gene expression is critical. Current research indicates whole, nutrient-dense foods (and exercise) have a positive impact on gene expression, turning on some good genes while shutting off some destructive genes.

Choosing a Healthy Nutritional Path

A continuum of nutritional programs follows, ranging from deadly to less-than-ideal to health-promoting. Of those represented, the Harvard is health-promoting, and especially the Fuhrman approach is associated with the prevention and reversal of heart disease and type 2 diabetes.

The Standard American Diet (SAD)

The Standard American Diet includes a large percentage of calories from animal products. It is high in fat—35 percent overall, including saturated fat. It is 15 percent protein and 50 percent carbohydrate, with many calories from processed foods. It is high in sugar, white bread, white rice, trans fat, salt, and unhealthy preservatives and low in fresh fruit and fresh and cooked vegetables. The diet is killing many Americans prematurely and plays a significant part in the type 2 diabetes epidemic.

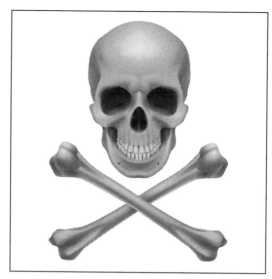

Research on the Standard American Diet's impact on children is alarming. Children are developing type 2 diabetes, showing signs of atherosclerosis, and, in adult life, an increased risk for cancer.

A Better Diet - A Recommended Diet of the ADA and AHA

The diets recommended by the American Diabetes Association and American Heart Association will slow the progression of heart disease and the complications of type 2 diabetes and are superior to the SAD diet. These diets will not, however, typically reverse heart disease or type 2 diabetes. Research conducted with Dr. Dean Ornish's diet showed a reversal of heart disease, while those on the AHA Healthy Heart diet experienced an increase in their disease (though not as much an increase as is found with the standard American diet).

A Still Better Diet – The Evidence-Based Harvard Recommendation

The Harvard School of Public Health's nutritional approach is based on current research without the food industry's influence. It emphasizes consuming fresh fruits, cooked and raw vegetables, whole grains, nuts, and seeds. Healthy oils are also included in the plan. The amount of meat and dairy in the plan is less than represented in the current USDA Food Plate. Red meat is especially limited. Bacon and other processed meats are to be avoided. Staying physically active is key.

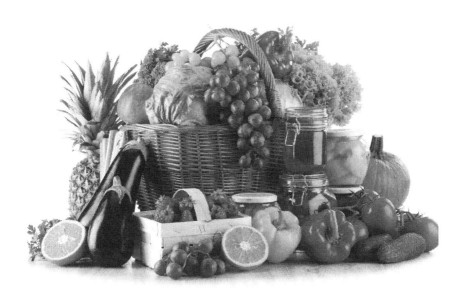

Walking the Ideal Path - A Truly Scientific Approach to Eating

The Nutritarian Diet, designed by Joel Fuhrman, M.D., emphasizes a whole food, plant-based diet. Dr. Fuhrman has incorporated food science information into an algorithm that accurately reflects the nutritional value of each food. As he has worked with patients and digs into the current research, he has built a convincing case for preventing and reversing major diseases. He explains his formula for healthy eating:

Health = Nutrients/Calories (H=N/C)

Adequate consumption of micronutrients—vitamins, minerals, and many other phytochemicals—without overeating on calories, is the key to achieving excellent health. Micronutrients fuel proper functioning of the immune system and enable the detoxification and cellular repair mechanisms that protect us from chronic diseases. A nutritarian is someone whose food choices reflect a high ratio of micronutrients per calorie and a high level of micronutrient variety.

For a wealth of health resources visit Dr. Joel Fuhrman's website at *www.drfuhrman.com.*

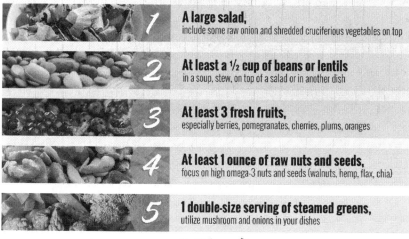

A SLEEP PRIMER

We Americans tend to be sleep-deprived people. Lack of restful sleep takes a tremendous toll on our bodies and brains, especially our brain.

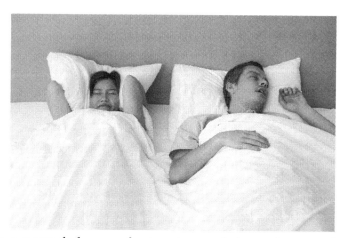

In a normal sleep cycle, two types of sleep alternate through the night: non-REM sleep and REM sleep. Vincent W. Havern of LeMoyne College outlines the normal sleep cycle as follows:

Stage 1 (Drowsiness) - When you first fall asleep, you are in Stage 1 sleep (Drowsiness). Stage 1 lasts five or ten minutes. Eyes move slowly under the eyelids, and muscle activity slows down. You are easily awakened during Stage 1 sleep.

Stage 2 (Light Sleep) - Next, you go into Stage 2 sleep (Light Sleep). In Stage 2, eye movements stop, heart rate slows, and body temperature decreases.

Stages 3 & 4 (Deep Sleep) - Then you enter Stages 3 and 4 (Deep Sleep). During stages 3 and 4, you are difficult to awaken. People who are awakened during Deep Sleep do not adjust immediately and often feel groggy and disoriented for several minutes after they wake up. Children may experience bed wetting, night terrors, or sleepwalking during Deep Sleep.

REM Sleep - At about seventy to ninety minutes into your sleep cycle, you enter REM Sleep. You usually have three to five REM episodes per night. Your eyes jerk rapidly in various directions under your eyelids, thus the name Rapid Eye Movement (REM) Sleep. The first sleep cycle each night consists of relatively short REM periods plus long periods of Deep Sleep. Through the night, REM sleep periods increase in length; Deep Sleep decreases. Toward morning, nearly all sleep time is in stages 1, 2, and REM.

Promoting a Good Night's Sleep

Give some thought to capping the day by meeting with God through reading passages from Scripture and talking to him in prayer. "I will lie down and sleep in peace, for you alone, O LORD, make me dwell in safety." (Psalms 4:8)

1. Avoid caffeine, alcohol, tobacco.
2. Avoid regular long-term consumption of melatonin. If you do take melatonin, take the synthetic rather than the natural. the natural, taken from animals, may contain toxins.
3. Do engage in exercise, but not within two or three hours of bedtime.
4. Regular aerobic exercise during the day can help you to sleep more restfully.
5. Don't eat close to bedtime. Allow two to four hours, depending on the size and nature of the meal. Fatty

meals take longer to exit the stomach.

6. Keep your room pitch dark. Don't even allow the light on the clock or DVD player. Blue light from the screens of electronic devices—smartphone, iPad, television—reduces the production of melatonin, making it more difficult to fall asleep and stay asleep. Use a filter or special glasses to block blue light. Avoid late night TV, working on your computer, and playing on your phone.
7. During the day, as much as is possible, have exposure to light, bright light.
8. Avoid over-the-counter sleep aids.
9. Go to bed and get up at the same time throughout the seven-day week.
10. Avoid watching emotionally-charged TV programs before going to bed.
11. Keep the bedroom for sleep and intimacy, not for work or study (or settling disputes).
12. Get a comfortable pillow, bed, and sheets.
13. Review your future "to do" list for issues or tasks that weigh on your mind or generate anxiety. Identify a specific day and time when you will attend to the task or work to resolve the issue
14. When you find yourself wide awake, leave your bedroom and find something relaxing such as reading till you feel sleepy.
15. Menopause and perimenopause are associated with sleep problems for greater than seventy-five percent of women who are in their late thirties through mid-fifties. Regular exercise combined with a whole-food, plant-based diet (tends to reduce estrogen levels), achieving a healthy weight, and sleeping in a cool room with light bedclothes and blankets can help
16. Resolve personal issues. "A clear conscience is a soft pillow."

If your efforts to sleep better fall short of what you need, consider talking with your physician about conducting a sleep study. Sleep apnea or other conditions may be the culprit.

WE ARE WORTH THE EFFORT

By taking good care of our bodies we honor our Creator: "I will praise You; for I am fearfully and wonderfully made; Your works are marvelous, and my soul knows it very well." (Psalm 139:14). If this is true, then how can we justify abusing our bodies, or systematically destroying them through poor choices? Our bodies belong to the One who created us.

> Do you not know that your bodies are the members of Christ? Or do you not know that your body is a temple of the Holy Spirit in you, whom you have of God? And you are not your own, for you are bought with a price. Therefore, glorify God in your body and in your spirit, which are God's. (1 Corinthians 6:15a, 19, 20)

> God pronounced material creation "good" and, after creating the first man and woman, "very good." "And God saw all that He had made, and behold, it was very good." (Genesis 1:31)

By taking good care of our bodies, we can better carry out our calling and our purpose. Body management through regular exercise, sensible nutrition, and restful sleep/rest is not an end itself, but it puts us in a better place to have the energy and clarity of mind to serve God across the entire spectrum of life areas: spiritual, relational, sexual, vocational and recreational.

Poor health is a diversion from what we are to be about. Poor health steals our energy and distracts our focus, preventing us from giving our whole selves to what God calls us to be and do. We cannot effectively reach out to others if our time, energy, and money are directed toward treating and managing preventable medical conditions.

Taking good care of the body promotes better health and fitness, enabling us to direct financial resources to building up the family, church, and community rather than for costly treatment and management of largely preventable, lifestyle-related disease and musculoskeletal injury. Time and time again, Scriptural teaching has much to say about money. We must take our financial resources seriously and honor God by using them wisely and generously. We know excellent health is more than a function of exercise, nutrition, and sleep. They are necessary conditions, but not sufficient conditions, for good health. A vital and growing relationship with God, solid relationships and intimacy with the special people in our lives, meaningful work consistent with our talents and passions, a clear conscience, and the ability to manage stress effectively are a few of the factors positively impacting our health

CHAPTER 8

WHO ARE YOU AND WHERE ARE YOU GOING?

One Dutch businessman, Emile Ratelband, age 69, has waved his magic wand. He has reversed his age by 20 years, so he says. He didn't feel comfortable with his date of birth, petitioning the court to change it from March 11, 1949, to March 11, 1969. Emile figured if people can reassign their gender by fiat, why can he not reset his age? He hopes the courts will legitimize his new chosen age of 49 years.

Putting aside all delusions, answer a question: Who are you? Do you have a clear understanding of yourself? Have you recognized your inestimable worth – your dignity – as one who is created in the image of God? Have you realized the unique person that you are and the aptitudes and talents you possess? Have you identified your life's calling and purpose? Have you come to deeply know, enjoy, and serve God and the special people in your life?

The answers to these questions are not found in the far reaches of your imagination, nor are the answers formed by personal decree. Instead, they are discovered in the real world by exploring what God teaches, how God has made you, and by acting intentionally to actualize what you discover about yourself. With a fuller knowledge of yourself, you can go to work to achieve an exciting vision for your life and the beautiful discoveries that lie beyond the inevitable barriers you will encounter. Consider the example below.

Years ago, Bill met with a couple in their home. As he sat with them, each described the emotion of emptiness. They said it did not make sense because they had well-paying jobs and lived in the dream house they designed and built with their own hands. At that point, one of their children passed through the room, and the father said, "And we have two wonderful children we love so much. They are great kids!" Bill asked if he had any insight into what could have contributed to their feeling of emptiness. Initially, they could not identify anything that stood out as the root cause. They began to explore each of the areas of life most people consider to be foundational—their spiritual life, their marriage, children, other special relationships, sexual intimacy, the meaning, personal success, and enjoyment of their work, recreation, and their assessment of their overall physical and emotional health.

Throughout the conversation, it dawned on them that they had inadvertently neglected the important relationship stuff of life by being so busy with their full-time work and the time and energy spent building their house. They all seemed at peace with one another, but there had been little quality time or true intimacy in their marriage and relationships with their children for a while. They alluded to their sexual expression as unsatisfying, indicating their spiritual life was nonexistent. They were living out what Charles E. Hummel wrote in his essay, "Tyranny of the Urgent"—that many of us are so busy responding to the urgencies of life that we don't take time for the important things. As they worked together, they began to have a clear vision of the specific steps needed in each area to reverse the emptiness they were experiencing.

How are you doing? Can you identify with the couple above? What would you choose to do if you could magically transform yourself in any way? Everyone, no matter how well they are doing, has room to grow; that is what we have reviewed in the preceding chapters. Let's review.

SALIENT POINTS TO PONDER

Building a Strong Foundation

So much of what we have come to believe about ourselves is drawn from other people—how we have experienced them and what their behavior and words have said about us. They are mirrors—accurately or inaccurately reflecting who we are. Healthy relationships require we not be at the mercy of whoever comes our way. We display wisdom when we surround ourselves with those who build up and create distance from those who destroy.

What we perceive about ourselves and our world informs and shapes our beliefs and day-to-day decisions. To be wise requires being able to separate the truth from the lie. Wisdom corresponds to the truth; acting wisely means informing and directing our actions with sound judgment. To be wise is to put what is proper and reasonable into action, promoting the good in us and what we desire in all we touch. In the first Psalm, we read of one who delights in God's wisdom and meditates on it day and night: "He is like a tree planted by streams of water that yields its fruit in its season, and its leaf does not wither. In all that he does, he prospers." (Psalms 1:3)

A by-product of majoring in what matters most is a profound sense of meaning and purpose to our lives, a deep awareness of our dignity, and finding an answer to the problem of our mortality and the inevitability of death.

An optimistic life outlook is sustained by a continuing awareness that our choices make a difference. We are not automatons at the mercy of our external circumstances. Parallel truths are that God is in control and, at the same time, our choices have a mighty hand in shaping our future and making a positive difference. The Bible does not explain how God can be sovereign and, at the same time, every day, you and I make real choices. Dr. Francis Schaeffer points out that the Bible teaches these truths from Genesis through Revelation but does not explain how. "The Bible states both and walks away."

Ongoing success in life means not going it alone. We need other people, and we learn from others. Going it alone is unwise, especially when faced with challenging circumstances: "And though a man might prevail against one who is alone, two will withstand him—a threefold cord is not quickly broken." (Ecclesiastes 4:12) Choose friends wisely: "A man of many companions may come to ruin, but there is a friend who sticks closer than a brother." (Proverbs 18:24)

Relationships

People are made for people, and the people space in our being can be filled only with knowing, enjoying, and serving others. No substitutes, please. Our health and even longevity are tied to the people in our lives. From infancy throughout our years, the nature of our contact and interaction with others, the depth of intimacy or lack of intimacy, whether others tear you down or build you up, and the maturity of character of those with whom we associate all are potent factors in whether we will fare well or fail well.

Who are the special people in your life? Are you getting enough time with them? Can you think of an important relationship in which a significant barrier has been erected? Can you take a step— for example, extending forgiveness or asking forgiveness—to break down that wall?

Knowing God

Our spiritual space can only be filled by a relationship with God— knowing, enjoying, and serving him. Again, no substitutes, please. Buford, one of Bill's fellow dorm residents at Clemson, seemed to recognize the importance of worshipping some semblance of God. Antagonistic to the Judeo-Christian God, not to mention the other gods of other world religions, Buford decided to fashion his own by carving a wooden idol he named Frigga. In giant letters on his dorm room wall, Buford painted "FRIGGA SAVES." Buford made no converts, probably due to the obvious shortcomings of a wooden idol and possibly due to a loss of credibility when word got out that he had accidentally shot himself in the foot practicing quick draws with a loaded revolver.

Except for the unique, historic, biblical Christian Faith, all the religions of the world, when it comes to their requisite for salvation, put their stock in doing—performing well, sacrificing much, chalking up more good deeds than bad, keeping rules, canceling out bad Karma with good Karma, etc. Christianity teaches that our behavior is inextricably tied to one's faith but as an expression of true faith, not the means of receiving salvation. It is the message when the Apostle Paul says that keeping the rules is not the way to go:

> Know that a man is justified not by performing what the Law commands but by faith in Jesus Christ. We ourselves are justified by our faith and not by our obedience to the Law. (Galatians 2:16 in the paraphrased version by J.B. Phillips)

When we do have faith, it is expressed in our behavior:

> Now, what use is it, my brothers, for a man to say he "has faith" if his actions do not correspond with it? Could that sort of faith save anyone's soul? If a fellow man or woman has no clothes to wear and nothing to eat, and one of you say, "Good luck to you I hope you'll keep warm and find enough to eat", and yet give them nothing to meet their physical needs, what on earth is the good of that? Yet that is exactly what a bare faith without a corresponding life is like—useless and dead. (James 2:14-17, paraphrased version by J.B. Phillips)

J. B. Phillips also wrote a book, *Your God Is Too Small*. His message was to those of us identifying with the Christian Faith. Do you have a view of God that keeps him on the shelf, basically inadequate to meet your needs and impotent in shaping the world around you?

J. I. Packer, in his book *Knowing God*, presents a clear statement of how we would have to approach the nature of God as presented in the New and Old Testaments of the Bible, a God who is far bigger than we can imagine:

> We shall have to deal with the Godhead of God, the qualities of deity which set God apart from humans and mark the difference and distance between the Creator and his creatures: such qualities as his self-existence, his infinity, his eternity, his unchangeableness.

We shall have to deal with the powers of God: his almightiness, his omniscience, his omnipresence. We shall have to deal with the perfections of God, the aspects of his moral character which are manifested in his words and deeds-his holiness, his love, and mercy, his truthfulness, his faithfulness, his goodness, his patience, his justice. We shall have to take note of what pleases him, what offends him, what awakens his wrath, what affords him satisfaction and joy. (*Knowing God*, p. 19. InterVarsity Press. Kindle Edition)

What is your understanding of God, and what place does God have in the world and in your life? Do you know what you believe and why?

The Christian life is not intended to be an anti-intellectual journey. There is a strong case for what we believe.

- Is the Bible we have today faithful to the original manuscripts, and how could we know? The science of textual criticism has confirmed that, for all practical purposes, we have the original manuscripts.

- Is the history recorded in the New and Old Testaments accurate, and how do we know? Over recent decades, scholarly examination of the evidence, including that provided by archeology, has consistently confirmed that the historical narratives of the Bible are accurate for the events, names, and places recorded.

- There are Bible historical narratives that not yet have been confirmed by archeology, and have been challenged as to their authenticity. For example, the stories about King David, his kingdom, his exploits, and the sheer numbers of soldiers and citizens reported have been challenged. We would say three things about this controversy. First, the narratives have not been falsified. Secondly, so much of the history recorded in the Bible *has* been confirmed by archeology, lending credibility to the narratives not yet confirmed by non-Biblical sources. Thirdly, the narratives contain such detail that they present as factual. As time goes by, more and more of the Bible claims and its overall credibility have been confirmed.

- It is fashionable to say that the Bible is historically accurate *except* for the miracles described. The miraculous work of God is so intertwined with Biblical historical narrative that you cannot reasonably separate them. Take, for example, the miracles of Jesus. You cannot remove His miracles without essentially eliminating Him as well.

What does the Bible teach about Jesus, and what does Jesus claim about Himself? The hundreds of Old Testament prophesies fulfilled in Jesus, Jesus' claims about Himself, and the claims of the New Testament writers present Him as God incarnate—One who is fully human and fully God. He claims to be, and the Biblical writers claim that Jesus is the way, and the only way, to Salvation. Recall, for example, the following Biblical texts:

> Therefore the Lord himself will give you a sign. Behold, the virgin shall conceive and bear a son, and shall call his name Immanuel. (Isaiah 7:14)

> For to us a child is born, to us a son is given; and the government shall be upon his shoulder, and his name shall be called Wonderful Counselor, Mighty God, Everlasting Father, Prince of Peace. (Isaiah 9:6)

> And the angel said to her, "Do not be afraid, Mary, for you have found favor with God. And behold, you will conceive in your womb and bear a son, and you shall call his name Jesus. He will be great and will be called the Son of the Most High. And the Lord God will give to him the throne of his father David." And Mary said to the angel, "How will this be, since I am a virgin?" And the angel answered her, "The Holy Spirit will come upon you, and the power of the Most High will overshadow you; therefore the child to be born will be called holy—the Son of God." (Luke 1:30-32; 34-35)

> For God so loved the world, that he gave his only Son, that whoever believes in him should not perish but have eternal life. For God did not send his Son into the world to condemn the world, but in order that the world might be saved through him. Whoever believes in him is not condemned, but whoever does not believe is condemned already, because he has not believed in the name of the only Son of God. (John 3:16-18)

My sheep hear my voice, and I know them, and they follow me. I give them eternal life, and they will never perish, and no one will snatch them out of my hand. My Father, who has given them to me, is greater than all, and no one is able to snatch them out of the Father's hand. I and the Father are one. (John 10:27-30)

In the beginning was the Word, and the Word was with God, and the Word was God. He was in the beginning with God. All things were made through him, and without him was not any thing made that was made. (John 1:1-3)

And we know that the Son of God has come and has given us understanding, so that we may know him who is true; and we are in him who is true, in his Son Jesus Christ. He is the true God and eternal life. (1 John 5:20)

Long ago, at many times and in many ways, God spoke to our fathers by the prophets, but in these last days, he has spoken to us by his Son, whom he appointed the heir of all things, through whom also he created the world. He is the radiance of the glory of God and the exact imprint of his nature, and he upholds the universe by the word of his power. (Hebrews 1:1-3)

Finding Your Purpose

We find a sense of purpose in our relationships and our work. We find meaning and satisfaction in the training and education that fortify us and equip us to do all we are called to do. The ultimate purpose is in a vital and growing relationship with God, being guided and powered by Him in all we do.

Paul Haefner was discouraged when he first moved into a nursing home in the Pittsburgh area. He was in his mid-seventies and had a progressive condition that paralyzed him from the neck down. He could no longer bathe, shave, dress, or feed himself. As to movement, he could only turn his head and move his left hand and wrist.

Paul was a loyal fan who closely followed every Pittsburgh professional sports team, displayed a compassionate heart for others, and had a sharp mind. His memory of facts, figures, and names was incredible. His dedication extended beyond the Steelers, Pirates, and Penguins to helping others. He said, "I cannot move, so

I have to have others care for me. I see others around me who can move, but they don't. They lay in bed or sit in a chair or wheelchair all day. I want to change that."

Paul discovered a tool for helping people identify their abilities and interests. He set out to administer the survey to residents and then interpret the result with each one he recruited to take the survey. Through their ability/interest profile and strong words of encouragement, Paul was able to stir them to action to connect with activities available in the building.

Until then, Paul had wholly depended on staff and volunteers to move about the building in his wheelchair. However, because of his new official volunteer role, his insurance carrier would now provide a motorized wheelchair. That left hand, still capable of movement, allowed him to operate the tennis ball-toggle switch on the chair and independently scoot about the building to visit his friends and meet his newly adopted clients. Paul aptly named his program "Potential Unlimited" and had business cards printed and distributed.

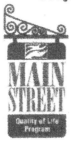

Paul Haefner (412) 625-1572
Project Manager X5780

Potential Unlimited
A Project of the Main Street
Quality of Life Program

Paul later became the chairperson for the Resident Committee and was the number one go-to person when the state annually sent in its inspectors. He actively participated in the many activities he had promoted to others—programs, games, having a character part in musicals and plays, participating in small groups, going on field trips, and, on rare occasions, attending a Pirates baseball game.

Paul continuously stretched the boundaries of his life. He had a strong faith and a sense of purpose. He knew he had an essential place in his world.

What about you? What personal talents, aptitudes, and passions can you put to work in the service of others? Suppose your primary work or occupation does not fully engage your talents and interests.

What contrasting avocation or serious hobby would complement your full-time work by providing an added path of expression?

Recommended sources related to strengthening your faith:

Already mentioned, *Knowing God*, by J.I. Packer.

Two fascinating and thought-providing books by J. Warner Wallace: *Cold Case Christianity: A Homicide Detective Investigates the Claims of the Gospels*; and *Gods' Crime Scene: A Cold-Case Detective Examines the Evidence for a Divinely Created Universe*.

The Holiness of God, by R.C. Sproul, and any of his other one-hundred books; also, other printed, audio, and video resources available through Ligonier Ministries, founded by Dr. Sproul.

Fortify and Enrich Your Body

There is a strong case—spiritually and scientifically—for being a wise manager of your body and brain.

Jon Kolb is a former All-Pro Pittsburgh Steeler who earned four Super Bowl Rings. He is an exercise physiologist who teaches at a university and works wonders with clients through his Pennsylvania-based organization, *Adventures in Training with a Purpose.* Jon believes many of us fail to sustain efforts toward health, fitness, and performance because we don't have a strong enough sense of purpose to continue. We tend to elevate goals above purpose. A recurring theme in Jon's work is to compare Being the Best as opposed to Being the Best that We Can Be. He says our parents, coaches, and teachers encourage us to be the best. That, he says, is destined for frustration because we cannot always be the best. But on the other hand, we can always be the best we can be. Jon directs our attention to a New Testament text that emphasizes our being complete and whole: "Now may the God of peace himself sanctify you completely and may your whole spirit and soul and body be kept blameless at the coming of our Lord Jesus Christ." (1 Thessalonians 5:23)

Are you as convinced as we are that creating and maintaining a strong body is worth the commitment? Are you motivated and dedicated to creating and continuing a healthy lifestyle path? More than ninety percent of adults who lose weight will regain it, and then some. Most of those who join a big gym drop out or diminish their attendance within three months. We recognize that all of us may have periods of struggle where we are less than enthusiastic. That's okay as we push through these periods and stay on track. Having a partner, working with a group, or having a designated person hold us accountable can help. Having a sense of purpose for what we do is even better!

Health Through Exercise, Nutrition, and Sleep

We have asserted that your health is much more a function of your choices than your genes, gender, or age. God has built tremendous disease prevention and recovery potential into your body and brain. As you age, you can only do what you train for. If your exercise is nonexistent, your sleep is insufficient, and your nutritional intake is poor, you will suffer the unnecessary disabilities and loss of independence too often associated with aging. If your exercise is limited to walking, do not be surprised when your balance, flexibility, coordination, agility, range of motion, bone strength, muscle strength, power, and endurance deteriorate exponentially in the latter years. Remember that seventy percent of muscle loss is not due to aging but neglect of participation in critical muscle-building activities.

What is your level of motivation to do what it takes to be healthy and fit? The Prochaska and DiClemente's *Stages of Change Model* is designed to help determine where we stand. Choose a theme—exercise, nutrition, or sleep—and identify where you are on the continuum of the six stages. If you are not at least at stage three, what would it take to have you step forward? What internal or external barriers are you encountering?

> STAGE 1 - **Precontemplation**: I am not aware of problem behavior that needs to be changed.
>
> STAGE 2 - **Contemplation**: I acknowledge there is a problem, but I am not yet ready to move forward
>
> STAGE 3 – **Preparation:** I am getting ready to change.
>
> STAGE 4 – **Action**: I am taking steps to change my behavior.
>
> STAGE 5 – **Maintenance**: I have made some changes and I am maintaining new habits.
>
> STAGE 6 – **Relapse:** I have fallen back to older behaviors and abandoning the new changes.

Emotional Health

We have proposed that our core beliefs are critical to our emotional health. Optimism flows when one believes our choices have a decisive say in shaping our lives. Take the second grader who had hit a rough patch. Each morning, he cried before going to school and had to be pulled away from his mom. To make things worse, the little girl in his class started calling him a crybaby.

That little guy's mom tried every approach—talking through his concerns, being extra nice, and then extra stern-- but nothing worked. On Monday morning, she told him if he could go all week without crying, she would take him out of school early on Friday for a special afternoon together. Guess what? He made it! Mom was trying to get him to stop crying, but more than anything, she wanted him to see that he had a choice and the power to make a . How much power do you have in shaping your future? Our core beliefs are a powerful force in determining our well-being.

A second factor impacting our emotional health has to do with closure. Emotional and physical health suffers when we carry burdens from the past accompanied by pools of negative emotion or feelings: fear, anxiety, grief, hurt, anger, guilt, shame, or disillusionment. The path to healing begins with identifying and owning the emotion or feeling, identifying its source—possibly with the help of a counselor, and determining the steps to take to resolve the root causes of our ongoing emotional barriers. It is good to remember that if it concerns another person, you cannot control another or their response. The key is what you do, regardless of another's response.

A third critical ingredient in personal wellness is the extent to which you are on solid ground regarding the critical areas of life. While emotional issues can sabotage your life in these significant areas, the converse is true: running on empty or stagnant in life's significant areas contributes to being emotionally unhealthy. A solid spiritual life, strong relationships, and finding your life purpose all contribute to comprehensive health.

This concept applies to many of those in the throes of struggling with significant psychiatric/medical issues. Without good cause, don't automatically count anybody out because of the nature or extremes of their condition. Remember Frank, whom we visited in a previous chapter—he freed himself from mental illness by taking one tiny step at a time as he took on each personal need, one at a time.

Years ago, Bill visited the locked ward of a mental hospital on the East Coast. In several hours, he had the opportunity to converse with virtually everyone on the floor. What struck him was everyone's life was completely on hold! The hospital's philosophy was, "Our patients are incapable of life. We need to medicate them and conduct therapy sessions before they can even begin to take the first tiny steps in pursuit of what matters most in life." There was no encouragement to move forward in life's significant areas—spiritual life, relationships, vocation, or recreation. There were no engaging hobbies or activities; they only exercised when they occasionally walked the halls.

Consider a different approach. For a significant percentage of persons with psychological issues (from mild to the more severe), the most productive path to emotional health combines therapy/counseling to overcome internal issues and barriers, administration of medication (often), and the individual taking small, but critical action steps toward fulfilling a life plan and purpose. For example, significant research shows that regular exercise may have the same or greater benefits as anti-depressant medication for some.

Another example—although it does not reverse or cure the disease—is with certain forms of dementia, such as Alzheimer's. Both regular exercise and good nutrition can help to slow the decline. For those in the latter stages of the disease, exercise can mitigate the acting-out behavior associated with it. We do not know how strongly it applies, but animal studies suggest that exercise can help break down the human brain's beta-amyloid plaque associated with Alzheimer's.

If a person is moving forward in significant life need areas, it gives them stability and greater strength to challenge and overcome their issues. We acknowledge that some psychiatric conditions require extensive treatment and medication and that progress may be minimal at best, such as individuals dealing with brain deficits, traumatic brain injury, toxicity, progressive disease-based brain disorders such as dementias, and abnormal brain chemistry or biochemically mediated causes.

No initiative or amount of effort is too small. If all you can do is sit in the corner of a room and wiggle your little finger, then move your little finger. It is likely that soon you will be able to move two fingers, and so on. Taking the first step paves the way to a second step, and the second step leads to another. Over time, self-efficacy builds (the individual's belief in their ability to achieve goals), cobwebs and dust are blown away from dormant abilities, and the person has the confidence to continue to move forward. Success in one area makes investing in additional life areas possible. With progress, an inner strength builds to take on the primary issues that led to the original diagnosis in the first place. Working through those root causes will significantly contribute toward the individual achieving more excellent emotional health.

Do you remember the most recent time someone asked, "How are you doing?" What was your answer then, and what is your answer today? One way to pose the question is to ask, "On a scale of one to ten, how are you doing?"

FINAL THOUGHTS

What did you get in touch with while reading through the book? Imagine waking up tomorrow with some questions: Did you have a good night's sleep? Will you start your day with quiet time with only you and God? Will you eat healthy foods for your meals today? Will you have sufficient and significant time with the people you love? Can you effectively communicate what you need and feel at work and home? Will you have opportunities to express your interests and talents? Will you engage in acts of service that will benefit others?

These are questions that we hope you will be able to answer well after applying the principles in the chapters you have read. Patience, commitment, and perseverance are required when identifying:

- ✓ Opportunities for growth
- ✓ Action steps for change: goals and target dates
- ✓ Barriers and resolutions
- ✓ Resources need
- ✓ Support to get the job done

Life transformation may also mean rocking the boat by doing things differently. Are you able to make changes, even if there is a cost? Are you willing to let others be uncomfortable if they become threatened by your progress and expectations for a healthier, more fulfilling, and more productive life?

Transformation is hard work, and we encourage you to be comfortable in the mundane. Achieving and maintaining a well-balanced, healthy life is often found in the day-to-day choices we make that, at first glance, do not appear to be all that impressive: the daily walk, eating a healthy breakfast, choosing to stop work and engage in meaningful relationships, recreational activity, and the time for thoughtful meditation in fellowship with God. Cumulatively, these steps are what will transform us into who we want to be.

In the book The Leadership Secrets of Billy Graham by Harold Myra and Marshall Shelley (Zondervan, 2005), we learn the evangelist did not appear to be headed toward having a significant impact on the world. He was extremely shy in grade school. His teachers could not get him to say a word. He was not remarkable or even memorable. In high school, he came out of his shell, and girls and baseball took priority over his work on his parents' dairy farm.

In college, he was messy and disorganized. At one point, Billy asked a young woman to marry him, and she accepted, only to later give back the ring. She didn't see Billy having any direction or purpose and didn't think they were right for each other. Billy had to face a harsh reality—he didn't have a purpose and wasn't going anywhere. After several months of struggle, Billy, while alone one night on a golf course, committed to follow God at all costs. Billy had some work to do in the following time, starting with his speaking ability—he was ordinary at best, but he persevered, allowing God to lead and direct his steps. Years later, one of his teachers saw him on television and couldn't help but wonder what in the world had changed him. The answer was God's work in his life, using his resources well and working at his craft daily.

We are not here to fill a space on the planet. We believe that God has each of us here for a divine purpose. What we do has the potential to make an impact, to be used by God for wonderful things—some of which we'll know and recognize, and some we will not know until Jesus returns.

Even your small, seemingly insignificant acts of kindness may have changed lives. In one instance, a young woman was seconds away from executing a well-planned plan for taking her life. But just then, the phone rang, and she answered it. The caller said, "Hi! I was just thinking of you and wanted to give you a call. I don't really have anything important to say. How are you doing?" That friend's small gesture saved her life, helping her to recognize that she mattered. Years passed, and she never again considered ending her life.

Where do you want to be in six months or a year? Five years from now? Affirm your life purpose and develop and execute your vision. Put your plan into action as you carry out all that God has called you to be.

> Now to him who by his power within us is able to do far more than we ever dare to ask or imagine—to him be glory in the Church through Jesus Christ forever and ever, amen. (Ephesians 3:20, in paraphrase translation by J.B. Phillips)

Blessings to you as you 'do life'. With ever grateful hearts, we wish you Godspeed as you continue on your journey.

Bill and Amy

RESOURCES WORTH DIVING INTO

We have published a companion guide to this book. It's title: *Your Life Your Purpose, Your Future*. It is designed for individuals and groups—to be used by itself, or in conjunction with this book, *REIMAGINE*. It is a guide for an individual working independently, as well as a resource for professional counselors, pastors, Sunday school teachers, Bible study leaders, and coordinators of church home groups.

There are so many excellent, thought-provoking resources to draw from. We mention only a few, many of which we have already listed in the book and are listed here for your convenience.

Dr. R. C. Sproul
> ***If There is a God, Why Are There Atheists?***
> ***The Holiness of God***

Dr. Sproul has written more than 100 books. Written and audio and video resources by R. C. and a host of other scholars are available through Ligonier Ministries in Florida (www.ligonier.org)

Dr. J. I. Packer
> ***Knowing God***

Dr. Packer is a British-born theologian who has served as the Board of Governors' Professor of Theology at Regent College in Vancouver, British Columbia, and considered to be one of the great theologians of our time.

Dr. Paul David Nussbaum
Dr. Nussbaum is one of the leading brain health experts in the nation, and has written a number of books, including
> ***What Is the Purpose of My Brain?***
> ***Save Your Brain***

You can reach his resources through his website (www.brainhealthctr.com/ and is found on Youtube.

J. Warner Wallace
> ***Cold-Case Christianity***
> ***God's Crime Scene***

Mr. Wallace is a Christian apologist and a cold-case homicide detective. He sifts through the evidence for the assertions of the New Testament, utilizing the same scientific tools he applies to solving a crime.

Dr. Douglas Axe
> ***Undeniable: How Biology Confirms Our Intuition That Life Is Designed***

Dr. Axe is Director of Biological Institute in Seattle. His undergraduate studies were at U.C. Berkeley, doctorate is from Caltech and he held post doctoral and research scientist positions at the University of Cambridge.

Dr. Stephen C. Meyer
> **Darwin's Doubt: The Explosive Origin of Animal Life and the Case for Intelligent Design**
> **Signature in the Cell: DNA and the Evidence for Intelligent Design**

Dr. Meyer received his Ph.D. from the University of Cambridge in the philosophy of science. He is Director of the Center for Science and Culture at the Discovery Institute in Seattle. His website: www.stephencmeyer.org

Dr. James Tour
> **He is featured through a wide range of podcasts, lectures, and interviews on YouTube**

Dr. Tour, an American chemist and nanotechnologist is considered to be among the top 50 most influential scientists in the world. He has more than 785 research publications, 130 granted patents, and 100 pending patents.

Dr. Charles Thaxton, , Walter L Bradley, et al.
> **The Mystery of Life's Origin**

Dr. Thaxton earned a doctorate in physical chemistry from Iowa State University. He went on to complete post-doctorate programs in the history of science at Harvard University and the molecular biology laboratories of Brandeis University.

Dr. Caldwell Esselstyn
> **Prevent and Reverse Heart Disease**

Dr. Esselstyn has designed and led some exciting research projects related to the prevention and reversal of major disease. His website, www.dresselstyn.com, offers a range of health-related resources.

Dr. Joel Fuhrman
> *Nutritarian Handbook & ANDI Food Scoring Guide*
> *Eat to Live*
> *The End of Diabetes*
> *The End of Heart Disease*
> *Disease-Proof Your Child*

Dr. Fuhrman is one of the nation's leading health life-style experts. His resources are available through his website, www.drfuhrman.com.

Dr. David DeRose
> ***The Methuselah Factor: Learn how to live sharper, leaner, longer, and better–in 30 days or less***
> ***30 Days to Natural Blood Pressure Control***

Dr. DeRose, scientific researcher, writer, and speaker, offers a wide range of health resources. His website: www.compasshealth.net

Barbara Arrow-Smith Young
> ***The Woman Who Changed Her Brain***

Ms. Arrowsmith was born with severe learning disabilities. Overcoming her disabilities, she completed graduate school and founded Arrowsmith School in Toronto. Her school is enabling children to challenge and overcome barriers to learning. She has been able to train teachers in her methodology across North America. Her website: www.barbaraarrowsmithyoung.com

Dr. Howard Gardner
> ***Frames of Mind: The Theory of Multiple Intelligences***

Dr. Gardner is a developmental psychologist and the John H. and Elisabeth A. Hobbs Professor of Cognition and Education at the Harvard Graduate School of Education at Harvard University. He is known for his theory of multiple intelligences. His website: www.howardgardner.com

And four more books for those who desire to put life principles into action, and desire to sharpen personal tools for critical thinking:

> ***The Wizard of Ads*** by Roy Hollister Williams

> ***Introduction to Logic*** by Irving M. Copi ***(very expensive bought new, but available in its 13th, 14th, and 15th editions)***

> ***Principles of Conduct*** *by* John Murray

> ***The ONE Thing: The Surprisingly Simple Truth Behind Extraordinary Results*** by Gary Keller (Also available as an audiobook, and accessible through YouTube)

Website for Ageless IDEAS: ***www.agelessideas.com***

REIMAGINE: YOUR LIFE, YOUR PURPOSE, YOUR FUTURE

The Authors:

Amy White, M.A., LPC

Amy holds an M.A. in Professional Psychology, and is a licensed professional counselor practicing in Butler, Pennsylvania. She also holds licenses in Georgia and Florida. She has served as a therapist in private practice and in both inpatient and outpatient clinical settings.

Amy has extensive experience in organizational leadership roles, including administrative and executive positions for non-profit agencies where she has served as a leader, coach, counselor, co-strategist, and educator. In addition to her writing, As a public speaker, Amy has addressed audiences in corporations, universities, churches, communities, and at national conferences.

William H. White, Ph.D.

Bill is an exercise physiologist with national certifications from the *American College of Sports Medicine*, *National Academy of Sports Medicine*, and *American Council on Exercise*. Theological education includes seminary coursework, and guided independent study. He completed his Ph.D. at the University of Pittsburgh Graduate School of Education, with a major counseling and a minor in psychology.

Bill's focus is to promote comprehensive wellness, addressing each major area of life—spiritual, relational, vocational, recreational, physical, and emotional. His avenues of service include public speaking, writing, and health/fitness/performance coaching and training. Over several decades, in addition to working with individual clients, Bill has served in the university, seminary, non-profit corporate, and in church settings.

Made in the USA
Middletown, DE
04 November 2023

41831790R00106